Bereavement Counseling
Pastoral Care
for Complicated Grieving

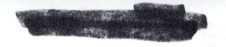

THE HAWORTH PASTORAL PRESS
Religion and Mental Health
Harold G. Koenig, MD
Senior Editor

Bereavement Counseling
Pastoral Care
for Complicated Grieving

Junietta Baker McCall, DMin

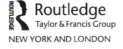
Routledge
Taylor & Francis Group
NEW YORK AND LONDON

First Published by

The Haworth Pastoral Press®, an imprint of The Haworth Press, Inc., 10 Alice Street, Binghamton, NY 13904-1580.

Transferred to Digital Printing 2009 by Routledge
270 Madison Ave, New York NY 10016
2 Park Square, Milton Park, Abingdon, Oxon, OX14 4RN

Cover design by Jennifer M. Gaska.

PUBLISHER'S NOTE
Identities and circumstances of individuals discussed in this book have been changed to protect confidentiality. Any resemblance to actual persons, living or dead, is entirely coincidental.

Library of Congress Cataloging-in-Publication Data

McCall, Junietta Baker.
    Bereavement counseling : pastoral care for complicated grieving / Junietta Baker McCall.
        p. cm.
    Includes bibliographical references and index.
        ISBN 0-7890-1783-0 (alk. paper)—ISBN 0-7890-1784-9 (pbk. : alk. paper)
        1. Church work with the bereaved. 2. Pastoral counseling. I. Title.
BV4330.M33 2003
259'.6—dc21

2003001808

To my sons, Jonathan Seth and Jeremiah Brierly,
who always focus on the possibilities that life has to offer.

ABOUT THE AUTHOR

Junietta Baker McCall, DMin, is Director of Pastoral Services at New Hampshire Hospital in Concord. A licensed pastoral psychotherapist and an ordained minister of the United Church of Christ, she is the author of *Grief Education for Caregivers of the Elderly* and *A Practical Guide to Hospital Ministry: Healing Ways.* Dr. McCall has served as an adjunct faculty member in pastoral counseling at Andover Newton Theological School in Newton Centre in Massachusetts, and as Associate Pastor of South Congregational Church, and has taught developmentally challenged children in the Chicago public school system.

CONTENTS

Foreword

The wealthy, powerful king had lain on the ground for six consecutive days and nights—fasting, praying, crying out to God for mercy. The ruler had not taken any food; he had not taken any water; he had not changed his clothes; he had not moved from his prostrate position despite the urging of servants and family members. As he lay prone, he continuously pleaded for the life of his dying little boy. On the seventh day, the king noticed those who were nearby whispering among themselves. He asked them, "Is the child dead?" And they said, "He is dead."

Thinking that the king would be even more devastated by this news, the servants were astonished when the ruler rose from the ground, washed and anointed himself, changed his clothes, worshiped God, and asked that food be brought to him. One of the servants finally had the courage to ask, "What is this thing you have done? You fasted and wept for the child while it was alive; but when the child died, you arose and ate food." The ruler replied, "While the child was still alive, I fasted and wept; for I said, 'Who knows whether the Lord will be gracious to me, that the child may live?' But now he is dead; why should I fast? Can I bring him back again? I shall go to him, but he will not return to me (Oxford Annotated Bible, RSV, II Samuel 12:16-23).

The man in the story was King David, a commander of mighty armies and the ruler who succeeded in unifying into one mighty nation the twelve tribes of Israel. Yet in spite of all his wealth and power, in spite of all his prayers and pleas, David could not reverse the slow descent into death of his precious son.

I have heard several clergy reflect on this biblical story in the context of graveside services for infants. The messages were well-meaning meditations designed to comfort the grieving parents with words such as these: "You have done everything you could to try to save your child. You have obtained the best possible medical care, you have been present in the hospital hour after hour, you have prayed and cried out to God. But now the child is gone. You cannot do anything more; now you need to remember your other family members, take food, and move on with your life." Although the words were intended to be pastoral and comforting, the message did not reflect the reality of the experience of parental grief. Yes, the parents may have been helped to know that they had done everything possible, that they should have no regrets. But the other half of the message—"get up, take a bath, eat some lunch, get on with your life"—withholds from those parents the essential grieving process of telling their painful story again and again and again. Rather than encouraging grieving parents to "remember well" (in Dr. McCall's words), the story of King David reinforces the cultural expectation that a significant loss can be assigned a defined period of time; when the "appropriate" time period is over, those who grieve are expected to "get on with it."

Grief is a universal human experience. The words of the Psalms, especially the Psalms of Lament, have echoed through synagogue and church for countless generations. In our pain, we sob and repeat sacred words describing the common experience of grief. "Out of the depths I cry to thee, O Lord! Lord, hear my voice! Let thy ears be attentive to the voice of my supplication" (Oxford Annotated Bible, RSV).

Yet in spite of its universality, the grief experience is also highly individualistic. There is a pattern to the "normal" grief journey, and clergy, clinicians, and hospital staff are familiar with the steps involved in that journey of recovery from major loss: *shock, denial, feelings, depression, reorganization, and recovery.* Dr. McCall's many years of experience as a clinician and a pastoral therapist provide her with a unique vantage point from which to explore these "normal" stages and then move on to an analysis of complicated and dysfunctional grief. In developing her models for small group work with those who experience complicated or dysfunctional grief, Dr. McCall draws from wisdom accumulated through years of listening well, learning, connecting, and providing a healing presence for those whose grief journey has become so blocked that they cannot move toward recovery.

> Complicated grief refers to a holistic grief response that is more intense than would be otherwise indicated; longer lasting than typical; and at the same time, pervasively affects the grieving person's daily life (and behaviors) in significant and negative ways. (p. 51)

When losses are so overwhelming that the complications become obstacles and eventually barriers,

> there is an increased possibility for dysfunction to intensify in the form of health problems, disease, and other destructive processes and behaviors. A barrier is built when a challenge or problem has become a complication or obstacle that cannot be worked through. The severity and rigidity of a barrier is what makes it a major criterion in a dysfunctional grief response. (p. 82)

Many of the complications that can occur are spiritually based issues, and numerous vignettes in the book illustrate vividly the spiritual components of grieving. Grief work *is* spiritual work because significant loss challenges an individual's core understanding of the meaning of life. When people access spiritual resources in ways that are negative rather than positive, the entire grief process may then become dysfunctional. "It is not the spirit that is dysfunctional, but a person's inner and outer expressions of spirituality" (p. 106).

Both pastoral caregivers and clinicians will resonate with Dr. Mc-Call's statement that the "primary treatment for grief recovery is talk therapy." Such "talk therapy" occurs in group settings where individuals can express their own reality and then experience having that reality "received empathically and validated as the truth for that person at the time of expression." In such an environment, isolation begins to diminish and connection begins to be established. In addition to offering the grieving person the possibility of connection with others in the group setting, the facilitator, therapist, pastoral caregiver, or helper must "convey a sense of confidence in the possibility of recovery and an ability and willingness to be a skilled guide and companion during the process." A variety of treatment modalities have been used to assist individuals whose grief is complicated and dysfunctional, but all rely—in one form or another—on "talk therapy."

On August 9, 1998, my thirty-three-year-old son Cory took his own life. As with all suicides, multiple factors led to his death, and the haunting question "Why?" can never be fully answered. The desire to understand is very strong, and the capacity to accept that which is simply not understandable comes very slowly. In my own case, an additional and complicating grief factor was the loss of a relationship with my grandson.

It was not until two years after Cory's death that I found myself living in a community where a suicide survivors' support group was available. As with other Samaritan support groups, the format for the meeting was carefully structured: each person was asked to give a first name, identify the relationship to the family member who had died, and indicate when and how this individual had committed suicide. There was simply no way I could have prepared myself for the searing pain of those introductions. Because confidentiality in such a group is essential, I offer a few descriptions that are very typical but do not reflect the actual statements of any real participants.

- My name is Patrick. My daughter Gloria hanged herself in our basement on July 10, 2000. She was seventeen years old.
- My name is Diane. My twin brother Tim died on September 8, 1997. He shot himself in the woods with his hunting rifle.
- My name is Luke. My wife Barbara died from carbon monoxide poisoning on December 26, 1996.
- My name is Laura. My son Ben shot himself in our garage on March 3, 1999. He was twenty-two-years old and had graduated from college the week before.

And so it went that first meeting with the dozen or so people in the room. Knowing I could "pass" was freeing, but as my turn approached, I felt an overwhelming need to bring Cory into that little circle. So, Kleenex in hand, I haltingly said, "My name is Carole. My thirty-three-year-old son, Cory, died on August 9, 1998. He checked into a motel where he took a number of over-the-counter medicines combined with an overdose of insulin."

I had spoken to Cory's death on other occasions because we had determined as a family that there would be no secrecy about his suicide. But nothing had ever been as painful as the brief introduction in that small group. The very depth of that sharing connected me—inextricably—with the others in the room. As the group moved into more general discussion, I heard someone express a sentiment that convinced me of my own need to return. The woman said, "You are the only people in my life who *never* suggest that my grief has gone on too long, that it's time to move on with life. You've been there. You know what it is like. You know how long it takes to move forward because a death by suicide has so many layers and complications."

June McCall's life work has been the development of a holistic group treatment process that takes into account those layers and complications. Her models support those whose losses are multiple, whose grief is complex. Her work offers hope for those who have found other therapies discouraging and futile. She knows that the one who is helping or facilitating a grief group must also do his/her own work in order for the process to have authenticity. She works from the profound conviction that disconnection brings additional grief while connection brings joy. She urges her readers to "take time to love life and to love learning about all of life. Then, take time to understand loss and to treasure relationships" (p. 300). June McCall illustrates her convictions by establishing a deep connection with the reader through the sharing of very tender poetry about her own losses.

As I work with local church pastors in Connecticut, I often tell my own story to emphasize the value of referrals to well-designed support groups. I try to emphasize to the pastors the importance—in their own ministry settings—of creating an environment where individuals need not feel that there is something wrong with them if their grief lingers. One of the values of Dr. McCall's book is found in its capacity to be useful to a broad range of professionals who assist others with grief recovery: priests, ministers, rabbis, lay pastoral caregivers as well as clinicians and staff in institutional settings. The book will add significantly to their knowledge and skills, and the spiritual insights will sustain them as they engage in this painful and vital work day after day ". . . I realized that, in lieu of a magic wand, the power I had [to heal] was caring, kindness, and empathy along with an ability to approach the situation with some knowledge and growing skill" (p. 306).

Dr. McCall offers us this humble sentence as the conclusion of her profound exploration of complicated grief. May the insights in her material contribute to your "knowledge and growing skill" in order that you, too, may be a healing presence for others.

Reverend Carole Carlson
Associate Conference Minister for Clergy Concerns
Connecticut Conference, United Church of Christ

Acknowledgments

At the age of six, I wanted to be a missionary and visit foreign lands where people would need whatever I had to offer. In the 1960s, I translated this goal into working for civil rights and against powers that promoted war and the proliferation of weapons that could be used for mass destruction. Twenty-four years ago I finally found out that I just wanted to help people live their lives with faith and with health. What I didn't know was how profoundly challenging and rewarding this focus would be.

Without the sharing and openness of numerous patients, residents, and clients I would have not had the courage to learn and grow in capacity, and desire, to provide services to those whose losses have been complicated beyond belief. I hope they are well and continuing on the road of recovery. I thank them for allowing me to walk with them.

I also thank the numerous colleagues who continue to provide encouragement along the way. I am particularly grateful to Harry Woodley, chaplain, who has co-led loss and recovery groups for over fifteen years. I am also grateful to Chris Hatala, psychologist, who was the first hospital colleague to refer people with complicated grief for formal counseling. Both of these colleagues continue to support my writing efforts and are good sounding boards.

Finally, I thank my husband, John Pearson, who continues to provide support as colleague and as friend. None of these books would be completed without his tireless editing and technical expertise. John does the charts, helps with the location of quotes, and even puts the final manuscript on a floppy disk. Best of all, he no longer fusses when I hand him yet another circle to be added to the appendix.

All my colleagues, family, and friends have provided wisdom and encouragement. They put up with the many production phases and with the limits on my time and attention during the frenzy of writing a book. Without them I would have less wisdom, courage, and hopefulness in this venture.

Introduction

A voice was heard in Ramah, wailing and loud lamentation, Rachael weeping for her children, she refused to be consoled, they were no more.

Matthew 2:18

A TALE OF TWO SISTERS

The elder sister was ninety-one the day she died. She had lived a number of years in a nursing home. In her last days she admitted that she was nearing the end of life and said she was ready to die. This was a brave conclusion for her, given her tendency to be fearful of change. I found myself a bit amazed because I had expected her to contest death and dying more vigorously.

Still, death did not come quickly. During her last six months many changes occurred in Violet's spirit and body. In fact, I began to really notice these changes in the early spring.

I had come to the nursing home for general visitation. As I entered the unit I heard a scream and saw Violet standing there poised between the nursing station and the blue chair she considered her own. Another resident was sitting in her chair and she wanted that person removed immediately. Both she and I were shocked to hear a nurse declare matter of factly, "That is not your chair. Anyone can sit there."

Nine months later, I looked back on the blue chair episode and on Violet's subsequent move to another unit. I remembered what seemed to be a quick visible decline in health and I wondered whether her death was just a matter of age and time. I also wondered how loss and change in her environment contributed to Violet's choice to die without putting up a fight.

Violet died in the fall. Her younger sister, Alice, died six days later. The day Violet died in the nursing home, Alice was in a nearby hospital struggling with pneumonia. Her condition was serious but she was expected to recover.

Alice had been moved to a group home four months previously. Prior to that time she had been in the same nursing home as her elder sister. As a result of this past move, the sisters were permanently separated for the first time in many years.

Alice lay in her hospital bed while I told her about Violet's death. She clearly struggled to manage the pain she felt as she heard the news. She asked for details about the funeral service and knew that she was in no condition to attend. She knew exactly where her sister would be buried. She spoke of the beautiful tree that would shade her sister's graveside in the heat of summer and stand guard during the cold of winter. She said that she would be buried next to her sister in that same location. It had all been arranged years before.

Several days later Alice spoke to me briefly. We had known each other for many years. When I began to tell her about her elder sister's funeral she became very quiet. Slowly she turned her face gently to the wall and away from me. She had never acted this way before. I knew then and there that she would die soon. She had made a decision. This was how she would manage her grief.

Alice died the next day. I believe that she had decided that she and her sister would not be separated in life or in death. Such was the bond between these two sisters and the grief from which neither one would recover.

Both Violet and Alice experienced many losses. The most recent of Violet's losses included changes in her accustomed space (chair and nursing home unit), changes in relationships, and even changes in processes on which she depended. These processes had contributed to her feelings of well-being and experience of safety. In addition, Violet had to contend with the loss of health and with the potential for loss of her own life.

Alice also had her share of recent changes and consequent experiences of loss. Some of these losses are evident in the previous story. Alice experienced changes in living arrangements, loss of closeness and connection with her older sister, the grief of her sister's death, and the concern for her own health.

Complicating factors for both sisters included the vulnerability of their ages, recent health challenges, problems that come with living in a nursing home, and the strain of relationships. Each of these changes brought experiences of loss and expressions of grief. The fact that the losses and changes occurred over a brief time added to their impact and made an otherwise natural grief response complicated. These complications provided the foundations of the grief responses that possibly contributed to each one's death. In neither case can one attribute the timing of death to "each one's time" without considering the effects of these complications.

THE DESIRE TO KNOW MORE

The grief experiences represented in Violet and Alice's story are more common than one might expect. I receive frequent requests from colleagues searching for resources for specific grieving situations that arise in their personal and professional lives. In addition, I receive similar resource requests from patients, clients, family members, and friends. These requests become an opportunity for consultation and for expression of thoughts and feelings, thus serving a number of purposes.

In general, people feel some relief in talking with a professional about their grief or the grief of someone they know. As these stories are shared, painful feelings emerge. Those who are experiencing grief ask questions about what is happening to them. Others want to know how to help people they love or patients, residents, and clients in their care. Students also wonder how to help those who come to them for care and therapy.

For those whose grief becomes complicated and perhaps dysfunctional, the need for help is heightened. In these instances, the painful experience of being stuck in the grief process is perhaps one of the most challenging situations that a person must endure. When this experience happens, life itself feels as though it is on hold or careening out of control. Sometimes problematic or dysfunctional behaviors, thoughts, and feelings develop and become formidable barriers to successful recovery. As these complications and barriers grow the chances of more permanent damage, distress, and disease increase.

The desire to know more about the grieving process has grown immensely during the past sixty years. Since that time research on grief has proliferated as has popular and academic publications. Grassroots responses, including self-help groups, have become more widely available with a consequent increase in knowledge about normal be-reavement responses. Still, we have a long way to go. Much can be learned about grief and even more be learned about helping people journey through it.

Even with increased research and growing resources, we continue to struggle to understand the processes of grief. Furthermore, many confess a lack of understanding of what causes this natural process to become complicated and some responses to be dysfunctional. Even though we grieve so many different losses and it feels as if we go through similar processes over and over again, we continue to think of grief as being related primarily to the death of a significant person in an individual's life. We are surprised to discover the complexity of grief that occurs during and after a divorce, when a job is lost, or when a chronic illness takes over. We have some resistance to under-standing that a number of losses can be just as painful and compli-cated as the death of a loved one. Often we are shocked when we are confronted with the crucial importance of turning to trained profes-sionals who specialize in working with grief. We continue to think that grief just happens and we should be able to get through it without help. Thus there may often be an additional feeling of loss about needing help.

Professionals have a growing desire for further training in the areas of complicated and dysfunctional grief and seek to know enough about grief to be supportive, make good assessments, and provide early and appropriate interventions and make timely referrals. In a re-cent psychiatric nursing annual meeting one workshop centered on dysfunctional grieving. In this instance both the desire and the need to know more about grief became evident rather quickly.

The workshop began with a brief review of the normal grief pro-cess. This is an essential first step in providing a foundation for the primary focus on complicated and dysfunctional grieving. After all three grieving processes were reviewed, there was time for discussion and consultation on case material. During the case portion of the workshop, Doreen, a nurse who worked with elders, wanted to know how to help older people who had multiple losses that resulted in a large amount of unresolved grief.

Sally answered that she asked elders to do life reviews and to focus on their accomplishments. At this point, one could see pained expres-sions on the faces of the other participants. In an effort to validate

Sally, the leader asked her when she would use this intervention in the grieving process. Her response demonstrated that the normal grieving process either had not been understood or had not been taken into account. Further conversation revealed that Sally had not focused on the assessment of "unresolved grief" and had assumed that the older person could "get over it" by focusing on accomplishments.

Even as other participants tactfully tried to confront Sally with her own denial mechanism, Sally insisted that this was the best way to go. She could not hear other opinions, nor could she enter the dialogue in an open and curious way. Sadly, lack of time and appropriate circumstances prevented an assessment of Sally's skill base or personal and professional issues that caused her to shy away from the pain and grief experienced by these elders who depended on her for care and help.

Clearly one workshop would not be sufficient to teach the objectives of learning to be empathic, developing compassion, advanced skill development, and use of self to facilitate grieving and intervene appropriately with those whose grief process had become complicated. While appropriate, these objectives could only be achieved by continued independent and concentrated efforts by participants. This workshop, although not meant to be introductory, was just a drop in the bucket of lifelong learning.

The leader, the participants, and perhaps Sally, left this workshop with increased awareness of the ongoing challenges of grief education. Still, the evaluations were very positive. Participants thought they had learned something and one participant stated, "I don't mind stretching myself when there is so much to learn." I thought to myself, "Who could ask for more than this—a desire to learn." With that desire much could be accomplished.

BEGINNING ASSUMPTIONS

Every author, teacher, caregiver, professional person, and clinician relies on theoretical and experiential frameworks that are rooted in multiple explicit and implicit assumptions. In general, the more explicit these assumptions are, the better the learning process and the better the outcome in terms of services provided. For these reasons the contents of this book are prefaced by basic assumptions that were generated at the inception of the project.

At its simplest level, an assumption is made that a need exists for a book that focuses on helping others manage complicated grief. Furthermore, this assumption carries with it several corollaries, each with its own derivatives. Each assumption and derivative is fundamental to the foundation and course that is followed throughout the project.

Assumption 1: Grief Is Natural but Not Simple

- Grief is natural.
- It can be extremely painful and upsetting.
- Many people struggle long and hard to recover from losses.
- Some people never recover.

Assumption 2: In Many Instances Help Is Essential

- Some kind of help is often needed to recover from significant loss.
- Help provided should be as soon as possible.
- Good help comes in a variety of ways.

Assumption 3: Training and Continuing Education Are Important for All Health Care Providers

- The average health care provider knows a little about grief and loss but not necessarily enough.
- The average health care provider does not have easy access to helpful interventions for complicated grief.
- A poor sense of timing and focus can contribute to additional pain and complications.

Assumption 4: Clergy and Spiritual Care Providers Could Benefit from Advanced Training for Grief and Loss

- People often expect clergy to be experts in grief and loss.
- Clergy and pastoral psychotherapists do not necessarily have advanced training in working with normal or complicated grief.

THE LARGER CONTEXT

This book promotes a clinical, pastoral, and spiritual care approach to helping individuals recover from complicated grieving. It is person (patient/client) centered and therefore intended to be practical and useful to a variety of professionals working with individuals in the depths of bereavement. As resource, or guide, it is based on observations, experiences, theory, and reflections of patterns of grieving, grieving problems, and possible outcomes of strategically applied interventions.

In contrast, recent literature in the field has focused primarily on normal processes of grieving, on grief nomenclature, and on the development of a clinical category for dysfunctional grieving. Grief and loss literature has been exhaustive in the area of normal grieving processes, but not extensive as applied to complicated and dysfunctional grieving. Frequently, notations concerning complicated and dysfunctional grieving are brief, with little or no reference to treatment strategies and interventions.

In the case of the ongoing nomenclature debate prevalent in professional resources, the interchangeable use of differing names for complicated and dysfunctional grieving has led to a lack of clarity in research and writing endeavors. Many names are applied to grief that is "other than normal." Complicated grief, abnormal grief, neurotic, traumatic, unresolved, delayed, and dysfunctional grief are just a few in a growing list that has yet to be sorted out satisfactorily.

Furthermore, numerous researchers have struggled to develop empirical data that would lead to an independent clinical category for complicated and dysfunctional grieving, thus turning it into a disorder in its own right. These struggles are often found in professional journals and have yet to reach enough agreement to be part of functional assessment and treatment planning. Meanwhile, professionals from all disciplines must find a way to structure current data within a cohesive and useable framework, no matter how tentative. Thus the larger context of the role of helper to grieving individuals is by no means settled or even structured as well as it will be in the future.

AIMS AND PURPOSE

This book identifies universal/normal grief responses, complicated grief responses, and dysfunctional grieving. It focuses on accurate assessment within this continuum of grief responses while recognizing that transitional areas within each continuum overlap at times. Helpful strategies are identified, to be used throughout the grieving process and specific interventions for complicated and dysfunctional grief are noted.

Ample vignettes are provided to serve as examples and to provide depth and life to the grieving process. These vignettes are composite examples and do not accurately reflect any one individual or situation unless otherwise indicated. Their purpose is solely to promote learning. As a learning device, these vignettes provide a solid and insightful learning format by helping the reader experience both grief and grief interventions in an experiential way, thus expanding one's own personal and professional realm. The expansion of experience is absolutely crucial in increasing one's capacity to help people as they journey toward health and wholeness.

More specifically, the aims of this book are as follows:

- To assist the reader with the task of helping others bear the pain of grief; process loss; gain new insight and meaning; and experience a renewed sense of healing and connection
- To be a practical resource regarding complicated grieving, based on current theory, observations, and experience, and inclusive of changing approaches and developing standards of practice
- To be a guide to the assessment and treatment of complicated grief by providing useable treatment strategies, sharing standard interventions, and promoting technical skill for caregivers
- To share narratives of health, bereavement, and healing that provide a living context for maintaining a people-centered focus, promote meaning, and lead to positive outcomes
- To further the integration of spirituality in the grieving process by focusing on the partnership between spirituality and healing, the resources of spiritual practices, and the functions of counseling and spiritual/pastoral psychotherapy

CHALLENGES

In the realm of complicated grief there are numerous challenges. Many of these challenges comprise the subject of this book as a whole and some are alluded to in the preceding material regarding assumptions and purpose. However, four challenges could benefit from more in-depth scrutiny. The first challenge is the personal grief experience and its paradoxical effect on categorizing grief responses. Second is a deficit of resources that speak to complicated and dysfunctional grief processes. Third, the spiritual component remains a predominantly overlooked and underutilized recovery resource. Finally, health care providers and other professionals continue to expect so-called "user-friendly" resources. This usually means that the material must be formatted so that it can be used with minimum time consumption and effort. This attitude is very practical, considering that timing is crucial to the response to complicated and dysfunctional grief and that professional resources are increasingly costly.

Challenge 1: The Personal Grief Experience

It is challenging to look at any human process holistically. We tend to struggle to see details and at the same time grasp the larger picture. We tend to know the here and now, struggle with the past, and be concerned for the future. This struggle is not so much a character or personality deficit for some people as it is part of the nature and experience of all human reflection and the human condition in general.

As Paul states so clearly in the New Testament in his letter to the church at Corinth

> For now we see in a mirror dimly, but then face to face.
> Now I know in part; then I shall understand fully,
> even as I have been fully understood. (I Corinthians 13:12)

It is our human fate and our tendency to see in our mirrors dimly. We think our experiences are the only such experiences. Thus, at times we think what we can experience and see is the sum of experience and sight. Such knowledge keeps us in touch with our current experiences but limits us, during times of stress, in our search for meaning, relationship, and context.

Apparently Paul knew the frustration of being able to see parts but not wholes. He chided the church at Corinth for thinking small and territorial rather than thinking large and finding a greater meaning in the present and in the future. However, he still tried to make sense of divine action and human behaviors. Even while leaving the full understanding of anything and everything to God, Paul encouraged others to grow in spirit, relationships, and behavior. We do likewise when trying to understand grief as a personal experience.

The task of learning about grief and helping others move toward recovery is one of those holistic quests that we can do only with inspired humility. Such is the case due to the admitted complexity involved in each individual grief experience. In general, no linear cause and effect applies to all people. No one intervention will work for everyone. We have no crystal ball. We cannot say with certainty that any specific loss, complication, or trauma will lead to a complicated or dysfunctional grief response. In this sense, the human response to loss is amazingly rich in resiliency even when it seems impossible for a given individual's grief process to lead to health and recovery. For these reasons, loss and its significance remains a highly subjective phenomenon. Thus, we must hold in our hearts and minds the paradox of each grief process being individualized, even when we presume to categorize types of response and patterns within those responses.

No one really expected Evelyn to become severely depressed. She had times when she and her parents did not get along, but everyone has those times. She attended high school and finished college. She was bright and well liked; she seemed to have friends and to take pleasure in her work. In midlife she drew on her respect and reverence for all of creation to keep up with her health care profession and with gardening, reading, and friendships. Then, over a period of a year or less she began to sense a separation growing between her and a best friend. She had been close to this person all her adult life. Now they fought, disagreed about everything, and even stopped talking to each other. Evelyn could not stand it. She felt that she was somehow to blame and became severely depressed. Her tears flowed unstoppably. A couple of years later her life was in shambles. Friends and family did not know what to do. They couldn't understand the power of the relationship that was now severed. The final straw came when Evelyn's friend said she no longer wished to see Evelyn. Evelyn's deep depression grew into an illness from which she would not ever recover.

Those who tried to help Evelyn began to realize that the friendship may have always been a bit dysfunctional. After awhile, everyone became aware that a full-blown clinical depression had taken hold. Few realized the depth of Evelyn's broken heart. To add to the challenge of helping Evelyn in her complicated and now dysfunctional grief, it was difficult to believe that such a bright person could not simply take medication, engage in therapy, and get through this. Evelyn, for her part, insisted that no one really understood her grief; she took total responsibility for the broken relationship. There was no happy ending, only tragedy. Evelyn became isolated, grew more depressed, and eventually took her own life.

This is where humility enters the picture. Each experience is unique, but wisdom must also gain equal footing, for patterns of grief usually can be observed. Making use of these observations is essential to recovery. This need for making connections during personal grief can be seen again and again in group therapy. Tom's experience is another example of the challenge to understand the grief within and the essential connections that must be made.

In the midst of a loss, grief, and recovery group session Tom, who is in midlife, says, "I'm a private person; it is difficult for me to share my feelings. That's how I was raised." Tom goes on to say that he has learned to talk and has found it helpful. He knows he must change his way of doing things when he goes home. There is no time to talk about his reorganization plans, for another person in the group says that her parent always told her to grow up, "like there was some button somewhere on my body that I could push to make that happen." Later on in the conversation she remembers that she was frequently admonished to stop feeling sorry for herself. She says she translated that into "stop feeling." The rest of the group picks up on the sorry-sorrow connection. The sentiment grows that recovery is difficult when one has been told to stop feeling.

Here, then, is a momentary connection between individualized and private grief experiences and the universality of all grief. In moments such as this, the challenge to assist in the creation of similar experiences of connection is seen and savored for its effect on helping foster the process of grief. This connective process depends on each person bringing his or her experience to the group process or to share with another person. Still, even with these experiences as foundation, the people in this group have a long way to go to work through their many thoughts, feelings, and experiences. Only when they have finished this task will they be free to make the changes necessary for recovery.

Thus we must continue to honor the fact that each grief experience is embedded in its own web of meaning. This makes tuning into the ordinary flow of conversation just as crucial as tuning into the dramatic moments. It is important not to underestimate the challenge of forever having to stay tuned into what is being expressed by another person. Such is the lot of a professional helper. Witness the poetically formatted reflections of a care provider during an ordinary therapy session with a grieving woman.

STORIES, STORIES, AND MORE STORIES

Not all stories are straightforward.
Today she began with a trans-Atlantic
wedding which led to a first holiday
without little ones;

followed by a house
whose ceilings are being repaired due
to winter's changing weather
patterns;

then pushing on to a roast
too well done on the ends
and yet, strangely so,
just right in the middle;

a quick turn of the subject
to insurance coverage
and other acts of a managed-care god;

while down below in the basement
slithers still the memory of a snake
suspected of bearing diamonds,
barricaded,
then boarded up
and smelly dead.

The truly caring and skilled helper knows the importance of staying in tune with each person while drawing on patterns, theories, and practices to lend light and direction to recovery efforts. It is always the case that this is more easily said than done. This is what places this challenge first and foremost on the list and makes grief companioning as much an art as a science.

Challenge 2: Current Resources

A recent search on a popular Internet bookstore produced 2,655 books available under the category of grief. Four were identified under the category of "complicated grief." At that time, none were identified under "dysfunctional grief."

What is one to make of this information? First, this kind of random search must be taken with a grain of salt for a more exhaustive search would perhaps provide other statistics. However, the information gained does provide a glimpse of what resources are readily available in the field. It also confirms the general state of resources readily available on complicated grief.

The current situation is not surprising. It makes sense to start with normal grief processes and draw conclusions about complicated and dysfunctional grief. This is, in fact, how most clinical theory works. We look at normal development and then move to developmental challenges and developmental disorders. We focus on normal functions of the body and then look at stresses and symptoms in order to understand illnesses and diseases. Even in the sacred texts of major religions, the sacred story is the norm for all other stories and encounters.

However, in the loss, grief, and recovery field the current challenge is to resist thinking that we know all there is to know because we have learned so much about normal grief. When such an attitude prevails, available resources cease to live and become codified in too rigid and limited a format. This must not happen, for there is still so much to learn in this relatively young field. Thus, a critical overview of resources for normal, complicated, and dysfunctional grief provides a more comprehensive context for some of the work to be done and the challenges that need to be considered.

Resources for Normal Grief

Extensive resources are found in the area of normal grief. Most of these resources are excellent and are based on theory informed by research and practice conducted over the past fifty years. Even so, it may be said that these resources have a tendency to paint too simplistic an understanding of natural grief processes. The stages, processes, and tasks are still thought to be somewhat linear and sequential. We don't pay enough attention to the length of the grief process or to the uniqueness of each person. Recovery is still considered as moving beyond the loss. Thus we tend to think that all grief processes have a storybook-type happy ending. We tend to believe that all losses can be resolved, with the proper help, before a person dies. Furthermore, we think these losses should be resolved, and the sooner the better.

Resources for Complicated Grief

On the other hand, not as much research or practice has focused on the field of complicated grief. Some of the recent work concerning violence, abuse and neglect, and trauma has provided further insight into the grieving processes that occur in the context of these experiences. In addition, further resources are needed to understand the clinical evidence that the death of a loved one is just one of the significant losses that lead to complicated grieving. By developing a better understanding of all losses and the variety of grief responses we will become better adept at preventing some complications and developing treatment strategies that provide better outcomes. In the end, all of us seek to have the most positive outcome for grieving individuals and to avert the potentially high risk of complications that can lead to dysfunctional grieving and significant damage.

Resources for Dysfunctional Grief

We need to separate complications from dysfunctional behaviors and be more precise in our assessments. As with complicated grieving, we need to follow up these assessments with more accurate treatment interventions. Furthermore, we must resist our impulse to have grief be orderly and predictable while still appreciating commonalities involved in the grieving processes. Grief is neither orderly nor easily diagnosed, nor is treatment as advanced as it could be. Thus we must always contend with a mystery that can be humbling to our most scientific urges to provide order and category. For example, we must continue to accept that a person's grief can be partly normal, partly complicated, and partly dysfunctional at the same time. At other times, we must admit that grieving can lead to health-threatening and life-threatening conditions and behavior. Finally, we must move beyond our protective denial and face the fact that grief can have dangerous consequences.

Challenge 3: The Spiritual Component of the Grief Response

Although an increased call for holistic treatment includes the spiritual dimension, much of this effort occurs at the conceptual level. However, even at this level insufficient attention is given to the role of spirituality in recovery. In addition, attention to the spiritual component in the grief process is not necessarily integrated into training, treatment management, and clinical functioning.

In some cases the lack of integration results from the spiritual component of the mind, body, and spirit connection tending to be less clearly defined than other dimensions. It is often presented in a language that is not familiar to some of the basic care disciplines.

These issues make working with complicated and dysfunctional grief even more challenging. As a result, professionals tend to use more clearly defined treatment interventions based on reconized symptoms and behaviors. This being said, the point is not so much that we need to focus on the deficits of treatment opportunities within the spiritual dimension. Rather, the acceptance of these deficits can empower us to make necessary changes for the benefit of those experiencing grief and for ourselves in our role of professional helper. For it remains a hope that, once clarity and communication improve regarding spiritual issues and resources, more sophisticated treatment strategies can be developed with greater integration of cross-discipline services to follow.

On the other side, those who are trained in spiritual care and pastoral therapy need to continue to learn the languages that apply to other care disciplines. These languages will benefit communication and collaboration as well as promote strategies that provide better outcomes gained from spirituality in general and the use of spiritual practices in particular. This development of evidence-based practices will empower people of varying disciplines to integrate spiritual practices more effectively in the area of recovery.

In summary, for spirituality to take its proper place as a component of grief recovery on a par with physiological, emotional, intellectual and social dimensions specific challenges need to be addressed. These challenges require that all of us take spirituality seriously and expand our efforts to work in a truly interdisciplinary manner in talk as well as action. In so doing we might just meet a growing desire that spirituality be addressed in all areas of life. Of the many challenges that a serious focus on the human spirit brings, four come to mind as essential to grief, loss, and recovery and are discussed in greater depth in the following text.

The Need to Confront Puffball Spirituality

The first challenge is resistance on the part of nonspiritual care providers and ambivalence on the part of even the most highly trained and holistic therapists. This resistance continues to be based on religious, social, and cultural values and choices. Resistance continues to be promulgated through continued popular support for the maintenance of a rift among spirituality, religion, and the rest of life. On the other hand, those who promote spirituality prefer to do so as a matter of faith and have little desire in making spirituality a tangible component to daily life. Furthermore, those who shy away from the religious aspects of spirituality are often opposed to theorizing and systematizing language and practices.

In sum, our society as a whole firmly believes that church and state should be separated. This is a sacred and secular belief, no matter what the specific spiritual, cultural, or individual practice. The challenge that this view presents is often subtle in its dampening effect on holistic treatment and care, for what derives from this belief is the understanding that life is real and has nothing to do with spirituality. With reality located elsewhere, what remains is a sort of "puffball spirituality."

All of us have supported this ephemeral view of spirituality at one time or another. In our own acceptance or lack of confrontation about the belief that the spiritual dimension is powerlessness to heal, we have practiced a form of puffball spirituality. At those times we believe that spiritual things belong to the thin air and change with the wind. We accept a general lack of truth, impact, and permanence within those things spiritual. As such, spirituality is not really grounded in this world and by inference cannot be proven and therefore cannot be treated. Thus spirituality becomes part of fantasy, wish, and whimsy. Then, because we conclude that one cannot describe the spiritual dimension accurately, understand its workings, or challenge it effectively, we cannot take it seriously. Poof! Spirituality is omitted from recovery efforts and this widely held belief hinders recovery and becomes one more complicating factor in the grieving process.

The Need for Cross-Training, Consultation, and Interdisciplinary Dialogue

Writers and professionals in the field of grief and loss come from numerous disciplines including pastoral care and counseling. Interestingly enough, a slight increase in dialogue is evident in some continuing education events that include spirituality themes. Since these are educational events, the dialogue is often more of a monologue and is again kept at some distance from the individual needs of providers, helpers, and clinicians.

Still, a crossover of serious dialogue on the job appears to be somewhat lagging, depending upon the organization and setting. This parallel functioning continues to represent the resistance and ambivalence noted in the previous section under puffball spirituality. Here it was noted that societal efforts to separate spirituality and religion have complicated the situation to the possible detriment of the bereaved. A continuing need exists for the advancement of a thoroughly integrated understanding of the role that spirituality plays in the grieving and recovery processes. This kind of understanding usually grows with exposure, consultation, and dialogue.

For example, one morning as I gathered patients for a loss and recovery group on an inpatient unit, a colleague stopped me. In one hand she held a small piece of paper. In the other hand she held a pencil. "Can you help me?" she asked. "Can you give me a very brief definition of the word "spiritual"? When I looked it up in the dictionary the definitions all sounded like 'religion' to me."

After getting over my immediate anxiety about the magnitude of the task, I decided to keep it simple. I stated with conviction, "Spiritual concerns whatever provides meaning, purpose, and connection in one's life. Religion is one of those spiritual practices that can provide meaning, purpose, and connection. Yoga is another spiritual care practice. So is meditation, and, possibly, going to the beach on a beautiful day." That's it, I thought, as simple and as profound as I can be in about fifteen seconds, and I continued with my task of gathering persons referred for the upcoming group.

Our brief conversation was very exciting. At other times I would have been asked to attend the other person's group and talk about spirituality as an "expert." That would have been fine and I might have thought no more about it because it is standard practice in situations where spirituality is taken seriously. However, the professional dialogue would have been missing, and that would have been a loss.

Even so, it is crucial to identify individuals who have expertise and to know the extent and limitations of that expertise. However, the separation of human needs and functions is for the purposes of conceptualization and management of specific and specialized needs but not intended to be a complete assessment of treatment of any one person. The more anyone of us knows about all the dimensions of human functioning, the better we are able to assess, intervene appropriately, and refer to those who can play their part in an integrated helping process.

The Need for Models That Include Spirituality
When Focusing on Health Care and Wellness

The first need identified under the challenge to address spiritual issues in loss and grief was addressed as a call to integrate spirituality into our social and cultural fabric. The second part of that need is to have that quality of integration occur in the training and functioning of professionals in the workplace. The third need takes us back to the conceptual work that needs to happen for the first two issues to be addressed. None of these issues can be addressed sequentially. Rather the process needs to be kept in mind as a complete process with differing foci that revolve around the larger challenge.

The crux of the problem of building theoretical models is a practical one, or if you will, one of praxis. Although the need for more integrative models is great, their development is slow. Those who have training in spiritual care and spiritual practices are not necessarily willing or able to devote the energy needed to build theories and models to support the practices that they have developed. Conversely, those who build models and theories are not always willing to give as much energy to the practical interventions needed by those in direct contact with bereaved persons whose grief has become complicated, and at times, dysfunctional.

I confess that I seldom hear a professional from any discipline talk about what model he or she is using in a given care situation unless it is in an educational setting. Even students are quite surprised when they find out that they actually have to come up with theories to support almost every decision that they make while under my supervision in a training program for therapists. This is because I want students to bring what they are learning in the classroom to their practice and vice versa. Eventually, as they move from beginners to more advanced interns, I want them to have internalized this way of functioning into their everyday practice and I want them to continue to promote and expect this kind of dialogue with their colleagues as a general standard of practice. In the beginning, the process is time consuming and often daunting. But the purpose is not to promote rightness or wrongness but to promote professional functioning within the uniqueness of one's task and one's professional identity.

Recently, I have been supervising interns who are working on master's programs in counseling. Prior to that, I had supervised and run training programs for those who were working on a doctorate in pastoral counseling. This new work with master's level students has proven to be quite a learning process for them and for me. In their case, they have a willingness to work holistically and to learn how to use spirituality and spiritual practices in their therapy. This coincides well with techniques that are a part of their primary discipline. They find it quite exciting to have this part of their training presented in ways that they can understand and with results that help them feel they are meeting the needs of the persons with whom they work. In my case, I find it challenging and exciting to keep up with therapies in other traditions, to learn what's happening academically, and to be able to present spiritually based concepts in a way that is helpful and promotes the greater use of these resources in counseling. The additional bonus is that supervision and teaching give me even greater permission to try to integrate theories, models, and clinical and pastoral practice in the larger context of my own therapeutic practice and ministry.

For those who do not have the opportunity to teach and supervise, other practices may provide the impetus for personal and professional growth in understanding and using interventions that build spirituality in helpful ways. The obvious opportunities are in writing for professional journals, research, clinical reviews, professional support groups, reading, professional workshops, and consultation. All these efforts require time and the desire to learn to reflect on one's practice as part of one's normal way of functioning, but the fruits are well worth the labor.

The Need for Practical Spiritual Practices Appropriate for Complicated and Dysfunctional Grief

It can be argued that models of grief and loss that include more than a nod to advanced understanding and treatment of spirituality are few and far between, although growing in numbers. Multidisciplinary models are even scarcer. More discouraging yet, models of treatment that deal with complicated and dysfunctional grief are extremely rare. And yet, the more complicated and dysfunctional the grief, the more essential the task of rebuilding one's spiritual belief system and consequent spiritual care practices.

It may be that what we need are individuals who specialize in understanding the spiritual dimension of grieving and of wholeness to do advance work on complicated and dysfunctional grieving. This advanced work could use a number of different methods, some of which are alluded to in the previous section. However, the most helpful way for coming up with practical spiritual practices is to learn from grieving people. They have so much to teach even when they are stuck in their own grief and feel they have nothing to give. Most people whose grief is complicated are highly motivated to use spiritual resources and benefit from a respectful and serious focus in the spiritual area. Simply said, it is not enough to think about it. One must do it, think about it, and do it again!

Challenge 4: The Needs of Health Care Providers

Recently, I was asked to lead a workshop on dysfunctional grieving for psychiatric nurses. I began my preparation for the task by asking psychiatric nurses what they would want to learn were they to attend a workshop of this nature. Most of the responses were formulated as questions. The most common questions that they had about dysfunctional grieving were as follows:

What should we say or not say?

At first glance, one would think that professionals who work with bereaved persons know what to say. Also, one would think that professionals who work with patients who are in the midst of acute psychiatric illnesses would certainly know what to say. Yet the concern remains. Thus our challenge is to learn what to say and to risk using our own voice in professional and caring ways.

How can we help?

The desire to help comes naturally to persons in the pastoral and health care fields. It is offset by the equally profound desire to "do no harm." When this question is raised the request is for concrete answers. While these answers are not the same for every person, the questioner assumes that the teacher, leader, writer, clinician, and pastoral person has some experience and has taken the time to reflect and distill information in a useable format. The challenge is to be concrete and practical—to encourage others to risk beginning the task of answering this question for themselves with our help.

How do we keep from hurting people further?

This is part two of the "how can we help" question. It is a sensitive response to the profound pain and sorrow that grieving persons experience during bereavement. This sensitivity is essential for helpers in the field for it is indeed possible to hurt others even when we have the best intentions. Part of this challenge is to truly respect that we can help and we can hurt and either way we have a responsibility to treat, and/or refer, and to care.

Just what is dysfunctional grieving?

The honest health care provider knows his or her limits. In that light, it is possible to be very good at many things and not so knowledgeable about other things. Furthermore, in the health care setting, there are other resource persons within the setting who are regularly called in to provide specialized services. Even so, the primary care nurse or the parish priest, pastor, rabbi, or spiritual elder needs to recognize dysfunctional grief in order to refer, provide support, and conduct follow-up services. It can be challenging to be in the learner position as a professional, but learning continues to be part of professional functioning.

What can I do?

This question is repeated time and again. Often a treatment response is needed ASAP. Professional persons learn to recognize this sense of urgency when caring for a person whose grief response is complicated and whose symptoms and behaviors can be readily identified as problematic. This basic understanding that treatment is essential and needs to be timely is usually correct. However, the question still remains as to what to do. The complexity of complicated grief and its often excruciating painfulness make it difficult to know what to do. This is challenging for professionals who want to "fix" things.

How do our attitudes and perceptions affect the people we are trying to help?

This question reflects an insightful understanding of the patient/ nurse relationship and its effect on treatment and healing. Again, the raising of the question is crucial to care and recovery. The answer to that question often requires careful examination of one's self and services provided. Taking the time to be aware of a patient's perceptions and one's own perceptions is essential for providing the best possible care. The challenge most professionals face is taking the time to do this kind of reflection and valuing it as both an effective and efficient strategy.

Can you give us concrete strategies?

Skill development is an essential part of professional growth. It increases comfort and confidence and often leads to better care outcomes. But strategies are best provided in an easily used format that is compatible with current roles and functions. Some strategies are easily understood and serve as reminders or refreshers. These strategies are often seen as common sense when actually they just "make sense." Other strategies are more advanced and may require teaching, practice, and a statement of rationale before they are used. In all cases, the question is specific and will only be satisfied by specific suggestions and/or guidance in pulling out knowledge that a person might not know that he or she already possesses.

Is it helpful to be upbeat and hopeful with people who are in the depths of profound grief?

This particular approach of being upbeat and optimistic while the patient/client is experiencing sorrow appears to be a natural response for some care providers. Often people who use this technique just don't understand why their perky approach is often met with sullen silence or outbursts of anger. At the other extreme, a professional may sink into the sorrow with great empathy and become just as depressed as the grieving person. The care provider's job is to be as hopeful as possible while being realistic. How and when to be hopeful requires experience and skill.

After reflecting on these eight responses, it is possible to determine that one of the challenges for these nurses is that they needed to know everything they could about complicated grieving.

What is complicated grieving?
How does it develop?
How can we treat it?
Why does one use certain interventions at certain times?
Which interventions are not helpful and which ones are helpful?

They needed to know:

How can we be effective in our treatment of complicated grieving?
When and how and to whom we should refer?
When to consult?
What are the risks and dangers of grief becoming overwhelmingly complicated?

In addition, to accomplish these goals and meet these needs, nurses, and all other caregivers, must possess or develop the art and the skill of being empathic. Empathy refers to the capacity to practice "feeling with" and "being with" the bereaved person. But empathy is not enough. They must possess or develop the art and the skill of being compassionate. Compassion, in this sense, refers to the capacity and the practice of "feeling for" the bereaved person. One must care for and about the bereaved person in order to be helpful. Clinical and spiritual care providers often draw on empathy, but its correlate, compassion, is just as essential in accompanying a person through the valley of grief.

Caregivers need to respond and act skillfully. They must be intent about learning and reflecting on their practice. They must evaluate and receive feedback about interventions and make necessary corrections along the way. Finally, a caregiver who works with bereaved persons must be open to the "use of self." The caregiver must pay attention to his or her experiences, current grieving processes, and the relational context of helping another person. Often this context can be quite intimate and almost always profoundly human and moving. In truth, the challenge that caregivers face is that there is always so much more to learn!

SOURCES AND APPROACH

The conceptual foundations for this book are based on biopsychosocial and spiritual understandings of the process of grief, the behavioral learning research about how persons approach change, and understanding how people most effectively learn following a loss that leads to complicated grief. To accomplish this the reader will be exposed to a variety of sources.

- The most important source is the voice of the bereaved person. These voices will be heard in story, vignette, and poetry. These voices do not represent real people but they do represent concerns, thoughts, feelings, and experiences that are common for grieving people. In that sense they are authentic without being specific. Some of these voices will be engaged in individual and group therapy. Plus, every attempt has been made to present voices representing a variety of ages, circumstances, and cultures.
- In addition, a review of loss and recovery referrals is included. Information gathered from this review will cover a ten-year period and over 800 admissions patients referred for group or individual therapy. Referral groups consist of adults and elders. Children and adolescents received individual therapy.
- The experience of parish ministry and pastoral care specialist students engaged in parish ministry included in this group are clergy consults.

- A fourth source of information comes from clinical work in pastoral counseling centers and from the supervision of pastoral counseling interns.
- A fifth source is colleagues engaged in chaplaincy in general hospitals, psychiatric settings, and nursing homes. This source will include some of the experiences of pastoral care students in clinical pastoral education programs.

All in all, the material provided in the book covers a wide range of settings and populations and covers more than twenty years of ministry, teaching, supervision, consultation, therapy, and learning. It is my hope that all these voices and sources broaden and/or confirm the experiences of the reader. In all honesty, what is most important about this book is the sustained emphasis on expressing the voices of grief, of recovery, and of the experiences of those who choose to help as companions and guides along the way.

OVERVIEW

Chapter 1, "Universal Grief Processes and Responses," consists of a review of losses based on a relational, contextual view. Within this context, losses can come from a variety of relationships and experiences of daily living as well as from horrendous and traumatic events, death, separations, and major life changes. Of particular note are the similarity between losses identified by professionals and those identified by the person who is experiencing grief. Within the context of definition and typology of losses the stage is set for presenting a model of loss, grief, and recovery, for understanding the grieving process, and for presenting the various grief trajectories that fall within the range of normal grief responses. The chapter concludes with suggestions of appropriate ways to manage this form of grieving.

Following the foundation laid in the first chapter, the second chapter, "When Grief Becomes Complicated," picks up the progression that may lead to complicated grief responses. The chapter focuses on the definition of complicated grief and on its identification. Stage-specific complications are described, as well as factors and information about those individuals who are particularly at risk of developing complications during the grief process. This is followed by a description of complicated grief trajectories, a grief trajectory worksheet, and an introduction to the grief response service wheel.

Chapter 3 focuses on "Dysfunctional Grieving." Once normal and complicated grief responses have been introduced, a foundation has been laid for the discussion of grief terminology and the labeling of grief responses. The desired outcome of this conversation is the temporary simplification of grief responses so that interventions can be made safely, efficiently, and effectively. In complicated and dysfunctional grief responses, it is important to be able to accurately assess the locus of impairment, the severity of impairment, and its current duration. As with complicated grief, risk factors and a description of those particularly at risk for dysfunctional grieving are provided. Plus, the grief trajectory worksheet is adapted for use for the three types of grief responses noted in these first three chapters.

Chapter 4, "The Spiritual Side of Grief and Loss," moves from conceptual material about the different categories of normal, complicated, and dysfunctional grieving and focuses on the underutilized spiritual side of grief and loss. Here the approach is similar to the earlier chapters in that definitions are provided, spirituality is placed relationally and contextually within wellness in particular and wholeness in general. The spiritual component of grief work is reviewed, as are typical grief complications which are likely to occur when one's spiritual side is in the midst of profound grief. The chapter ends with the identification of persons particularly at risk for spiritually based complications and with examples of these complications.

The next chapter, "How Perceptions, Thoughts, and Beliefs Influence Care," provides a much-needed bridge between research, theory, and treatment strategies and interventions. This chapter focuses on how perceptions, thoughts, and beliefs influence care and help others manage complicated grief. Myths and misperceptions of the grieving individual and professional and nonprofessional helpers are explored. In many cases these myths and perceptions have problematic implications for recovery. However, as is often the case, beliefs and perceptions can also be used to enhance care and increase the chances for a more successful recovery. For these reasons, the use of perceptions, thoughts, and beliefs to enhance care are given careful attention in this chapter.

One of the challenges of grief work is the successful building of models and integration of theories in the practice of professional helpers. Chapter 6, "Therapies and Treatment Priorities," is designed to aid in this integration by describing specific therapies and their place in the treatment of complicated and dysfunctional grief. A treatment priority scale is provided that is simple, but essential, in its format and usability. In addition, the primary grief recovery task of remembering well is addressed. Remembering well will promote a sense of continuity of being that can lead to improved quality of life.

Chapter 7, "Positive Strategies and Helpful Interventions," is intended to be very practical. As such, it is presented through holistic clusters that make up the essential content of grief and recovery. This approach is used purposefully so that the small picture, which includes specific strategies and interventions, can be fully integrated within the larger tasks that need to be accomplished during the grieving process. Attention focuses on working with typical and unhelpful grief responses that are commonly presented in therapeutic situations and in situations that require professional interventions. Finally, strategies and interventions for working with complicated and dysfunctional grief are also presented in a stage-specific format. The reader is encouraged to add individual experiences and expertise to any of these suggestions.

Chapter 8, "Reorganization and Reclaiming One's Life," provides a parallel process for those who have been working with grief as helpers and as persons who probably have their own painful grief experiences. This stage of grief has a chapter in its own right because reorganization is the most challenging stage for those whose grief is complicated. Helping an individual move toward being able to make a decision to reorganize after a significant loss is no small task.

For these reasons, particular attention is paid to change, and the stages of change, that are a part of recovery. Important material is presented concerning what motivates people to change or reorganize, the experiences that seem to be part of decisions to reorganize, and those decisions that typically challenge efforts to reorganize. Finally, the actual skills needed to reorganize are addressed, along with successful ways to help individuals understand that new skills development and change are essential to life as well as to loss. Particular attention is paid to helping those who experience failure, relapses, and problems that tend to lower confidence and cause them to return to earlier stages of grief.

There is much to learn. Thus, this project is somewhat of a whirl-wind tour of working with complicated grief. This book does not have the last word on the subject. However, I hope it provides good information and companionship as the reader brings individual thoughts to the process of listening, reading, and making changes in his or her practice and vocation. Most important is the intensity of caring, the desire for connection, and the willingness to reflect and grow. In that sense, I look forward to the continued dialogue that this book helps to foster.

Chapter 1

Universal Grief Processes and Responses

Often there is great relief in being able to put into words the
quality or the nuance of need and suffering. To suffer in dumb
silence, to be able to find no word capable of voicing what is being experienced, seems degrading to the self because it pushes
the individual back into a vast feeling continuum . . .

Thurman, 1976, p. 22

IN EVERY LIFE THERE IS GAIN AND LOSS

A middle-aged woman dropped by my office. She asked how
things were going and then began to talk about her mother.

My mother has Alzheimer's. There's always so much to learn. I
read books. I know my grandmother who is 101 could die any
time. I think we're prepared for that. I know my mother doesn't
remember that my father is dead. I guess we all have times
where we are still grieving. But it's not that heavy sort of grieving that is constant and goes on all day. I know, in this place
where my mother is, there is a staff person taking it hard because
a person he really cared about had a DNR order and he had to
just watch this patient die. We don't think about the effects such
an order has on the staff. As families, I guess we just think
they're trained to deal with it. They say you're not supposed to
get close to the people you care for—but you do.

During one brief encounter, this woman identified four experiences of loss: her mother's situation, her grandmother's potential
death, the death of her father, and the grieving of another caregiver.

29

She speaks of her own grief process and that of her family. She talks of grieving as a process. She understands that it helps for her to know more about grief and about the types of losses she and her loved ones face. She alludes to the roles and response of those who care for people such as her loved one. She anticipates future decisions that may need to be made. She is engaged in grief and in anticipatory grieving. A significant part of her grief work is accomplished through the telling of her story. This she does with a certain confidence, thoughtfulness, and simplicity. Her brief comments are really the summation of a lot of grieving that she has already done. She has had both support and opportunity to talk about her grief. If all goes well, the grieving processes for this woman and her family will be uncomplicated even though they are sure to have their painful aspects.

This middle-aged woman's grief story reminds all of us that every life has its moments of loss and moments of gain. When an experience feels good that moment is considered a plus and is placed in the gain column. When an experience is wonderful that moment is cause for celebration. However, some gains don't come easy and leave us with uncertainty as to whether we have gained anything. In these cases the gain may be that we have "held our own." One has gains in life when one is doing well, OK, when one is holding one's own on a tough day, or anticipating a good or even better future.

Furthermore, life's gains are valued for the increased quality and pleasure they contribute to our lives. Thus, gains are often experienced as moments or points of connection. Likewise, connectedness is experienced when important things come together in a pleasing way. Gain is realized when one is connected to oneself, one's needs, one's dreams, and one's future. Gain is realized when one is connected to people, things, ideas, and organizations to which one wishes to be connected. This reflection and valuing of connections comes from a process known as relational thinking and feeling. The process is natural because it represents the essence of what it means to be human, which is to be involved in relational processes.

Most people naturally think and act in relational ways despite being conscious of doing so or of being good at it. But not all relationships are equally valued. Each relationship, whether to person, object, or idea, can be of greater or lesser significance depending on the individual and the context within which the individual is currently living. This is the contextual part of a relational/contextual view of life.

All this having been said, nothing is particularly new or revolutionary about the idea that losses and gains are both part of life. However, in a time of loss this particular connection or worldview seems to be the first piece of knowledge to become lost or hidden as grief takes hold. Thus loss either catches us by surprise or confirms another crisis driven view that one loss often follows another or that losses are often greater than gains.

Still, the idea that life has a balance and rhythm that includes gains and losses has been known since the beginning of time. Ancient literature and symbolism have passed this belief to us in numerous ways. For example, the master of rhythm and balance, Ecclesiastes, wrote, "In the day of prosperity be joyful, and in the day of adversity consider . . ." (7: 14a).

In the early days of so-called new and scientific thinking, another illustration to the connection between opposites was offered in the discovery that for every action there is an equal and opposite reaction. This connective polarity was reformulated by twentieth-century behavioral psychology research through the demonstration that behavioral stimulus is followed by behavioral response and vice versa. Of course, ancient spiritual traditions also focused on the yin and yang of life. These are just a few samples used to demonstrate that idea of balance is deeply rooted in human thinking.

Thus, with all humility, the statement is made that every human life experiences both gains and losses. During our gains or prosperity we are usually joyful. During our losses we grieve or take time to consider what has happened and what it all means. It is this balance of celebration and sorrow that helps us retain perspective when loss occurs.

A RELATIONAL/CONTEXTUAL VIEW OF ATTACHMENTS AND LOSS

So, a relational, contextual view of life begins with the basic assumption that human beings are relational by nature. From our very beginnings we are part of a wider relational context and we are dependent on people and environment to survive. The instinct to be connected for the purposes of meeting a variety of needs develops in-utero and continues throughout life. However, we are connected not only to people but also to objects, things, ideas, and dreams. Existentially speaking, we are connected to all that is.

However, some connections are more essential than others. Some connections seem to clutter our lives and others seem burdensome and present obstacles to who we are and the way we want to be. Sometimes we purposely cut ourselves off from such troublesome connections and may even feel pretty good about those cutoffs. Often this is because we are the ones who make the decision to separate so the choice is ours. Still, other connections are positive and/or meet at least some of our needs. When these connections are cut off, even by our own choice, we experience loss.

Life Attachments and Connections

According to relational thinking, attachment is a state of being connected to a person, place, thing, experience or idea. The state of "being attached" involves at least one or more aspects of our self. We can be physically, emotionally, socially, intellectually, or mentally attached. We can also be spiritually attached. We can be attached through past, present, and hoped-for experiences and expectations.

Sometimes a physical attachment can be seen clearly. For example I am attached to my car. I like it. I need it. I still owe the bank for it so I also have a financial and emotional attachment to it. It connects me with people, places, and things so it is literally a vehicle for socialization and the meeting of spiritual needs. I feel I would be lost without it. My grief would be great if I were permanently without a reliable car parked in my garage and available to meet my needs.

Likewise, I have an even closer physical attachment to my eyes and all the parts of my body. I am also physically attached to the white damask tablecloth that my mother gave me years ago. I may not be as attached to the tablecloth as I am to my eyes but nevertheless the tablecloth and I are connected through memory and through the pleasure of physical touch and use. Furthermore, I am physically, sometimes intermittently, attached to other people. In the broadest sense, physical attachments are both concrete, and at the same time, extensions of thoughts, feelings, beliefs, and memories that are valued.

In addition to physical attachments some attachments are primarily emotional in energy. Often it is difficult to know how to label emotional attachments because we usually become attached to physical things, thoughts, and other people. Yet, I love the mountains of the northern tier of Pennsylvania. I remember the streams, the haylofts, and the potato fields of my youth. I remember the smell of fresh milk being processed in tall metal milk cans. I am emotionally attached to that area even though I have not lived there since age ten. I am attached to the wonderful feeling of love that I have in these contexts. I return to the place of my youth, to circumstances that remind me of my youth, just to experience the love and joy that I feel in those situations.

There are also spiritual attachments. I love the spiritual care practices of my youth. The smells of the sanctuary, the candlelight, the verses of scripture memorized, the hymns sung, and the people crowded in pews. I treasure the dark starry night and the thoughts of a God somewhere "out there" looking out for me.

We also have intellectual attachments. These attachments are to talents, skills, and ideas. Currently I am intellectually, emotionally, and spiritually attached to writing this book. The exercise of using my brain to put together a product that can be helpful to others helps me connect socially, emotionally, and spiritually. It also makes my mind work overtime. So the writing of this book, or the preparation of a sermon, or a clinical case, are of value for me and I would grieve were I to lose the ability to make these types of connections.

In another vein, I'm quite intellectually attached to the idea of "equality for all." I like to focus on the impact of choices on individuals. I appreciate all efforts made to help those who are oppressed and marginalized. I belong to a church whose strengths are inclusivity, diversity, and social responsibility. This concept is crucial to informing my actions and choices. While inclusivity for all is an ideal, it nevertheless drives my thinking, my spiritual quest, social action, and emotional responses.

Finally, all of us make social attachments. I like to be around certain people. There are groups that share hobbies that I like, and close family and friends. There are acquaintances. There are strangers in this global earthen village whose quality of life is important to me. I write to a young girl in South Dakota occasionally and support her through the Christian Children's Fund. Even though I may never meet this young girl I am now a part of her social world and she is a part of mine.

Everyone has numerous attachments that make up the web of reality of life. These attachments, connections, and relationships help to define and shape who we are. Plus, we define and shape who they are. We are interdependent by choice and by circumstance. When any positive or needed attachment, connection, or relationship is threatened, or becomes separated, or unattached, we experience loss. We respond by grieving.

Losses and Separations

In reality, life never stands still. It is filled with movement, energy, and direction. It is a never-ending experience of connecting and disconnecting. The result is experiences of attachment and connections and of loss and separations. Loss is an experience within whose context there is always grief. Loss is a separation and disconnection that happens in the process of living an ordinary day. We lose our keys. We miss the bus. We lose weight. We lose a parent. We lose our dream of what we want to accomplish in a given day, year, or lifetime. We lose our enthusiasm for the work we do. We lose our connection with God or our Higher Power. We lose the will to live.

We experience loss when we become separated from that which we care about or to which we were attached. We become divorced. We lose our home, our finances change, our relationships change, and we lose the identity we have had sometimes for years. Our children grow up. Tragedy strikes our beloved country. Four family members die in one month. All these experiences are losses and separations. Thus, we grieve.

New and Renewed Attachments and Connections

Yet, amazingly enough, life strives for balance so it continuously seeks new experiences and the renewal of the state of connectedness. These new attachments and connections are not the same as the old ones. Nevertheless, these experiences are experiences of recovery. If loss has to do with the connections we have, and the separations that occur, then recovery has to do with those experiences and connections that are coming our way. Unless our grief is complicated or dysfunctional, by the time we have grieved for a while we look forward to recovery, new or renewed connections with people, to different things, and to more ideas to care about. That is, unless we have not finished the work of moving on from the losses of what we valued before. The future life of connection is very influenced and even dependent on the past work of grief.

Right now, this probably sounds simplistic, but it is amazing how often I find myself telling a colleague that a grieving person's sorrow is very real because the person experiences disconnection, separation, and loss from a former connection. It is not our job to question the loss or the grief, but it is our job to learn more about it and the effect that these connections and losses have on one's life. If we could just remember this fact of connection, loss, and desired reconnection we would be much better helpers.

In summary, life is full of losses and gains. It is full of attachments and separations. Some losses are more significant than others. In the following survey of people referred for grief therapy, professional health care providers identified numerous losses.

TYPES OF LOSSES

One of the challenges in helping people get through losses is the popular misconception that a truly important loss occurs because of death. All else is considered to pale in comparison. So, when people are referred for therapy, they often begin by saying that no one close to them has died recently so they wonder why they have been referred for loss and recovery. Once a description is provided of the types of losses that people face, and may be grieving, the person usually takes a deep breath, a look of understanding comes over his or her face, and a list is offered of the losses that hurt the most. Often there are numerous losses. Frequently the losses given are not the same losses listed in the referral process. Yet there is usually a list of losses, for in cases of complicated grieving seldom is just one significant loss the cause for current grief. Such was Susan's experience.

Susan talked of her family. She spoke of doing two jobs and of having to manage a challenging nuclear and extended family. She spoke of several deaths that had occurred during the same month the year before. But, she said, with a big sigh and tear-filled eyes, "The loss that hurts the most is the loss of my job."

It took Susan several therapy sessions to state this feeling so clearly. She had been referred for group therapy because of the multiple deaths in her extended family. So it made sense to her to focus on these losses. In therapy she learned about the stages of grief and she heard about the grief that others were experiencing. She thought about her own experiences using the information gained in this group. Then she began to talk about other losses relating to hopes, intimacy, and general disappointment. She spoke of physical changes and their impact on her life. Four sessions later she came to the conclusion that she was stuck in her feelings of rage about having been fired from the job she loved the most and had worked so hard to get.

People like Susan can teach us a lot about grief and about the losses that precipitate it. In doing so they remind us to make our initial assessments based on as broad an understanding of loss as possible. They also remind us that we must accept and respect each loss as the very real experience of the grieving person. Our openness to looking at all of a person's losses and the grief surrounding each loss can help the person and us develop a much better understanding of what is happening in this individual's life.

Of two predominant ways to find out about the losses in a person's life, the preferred way is to ask the person directly. A less accurate way is to gather loss information from family, friends, and other sources. The following losses are a combination of both. By reviewing professional referrals for grief and loss therapy, one is able to gain a broader understanding of types of losses as reported to professional health care providers. This approach increases awareness and sensitivity. This approach can also provide an additional benefit of increasing the awareness of others. By increasing one's understanding about types of loss one is better prepared to know how to help people make their own identifications.

Naming losses is the first step in grief work. Naming losses accurately promotes recovery. Failure to identify a loss can lead to complications and inadequacy of treatment no matter how sophisticated the professional involved. Such was the case in a review of the discharge process of a patient. In this case, Keith was given an opportunity to go home several times for brief visits prior to discharge. Finally, he was discharged and able to stay home briefly before he was readmitted. The treatment team discussed his return. One person stated that Keith did not want to leave the hospital and thus his return. Everyone looked as though they agreed with this reasoning and no more was said until the grief therapist stated that she had just processed what happened with Keith and felt that a secondary grieving process was involved. Further, she explained that she and the patient realized that leaving the safety of the hospital setting where he had not experienced debilitating symptoms was a loss to Keith. This loss would require grief resolution just as earlier losses for which he had been referred. Once the team heard Keith's discharge described as a loss with its own grief they were better able to recognize that they too were grieving their own loss of having Keith return as an impatient. By minimizing Keith's grief they were denying their own. By honoring Keith's grief they could also talk about their own.

Types of Losses As Identified by Referral Sources

In the following pages types of losses are listed using several sources of information. A possible drawback of the review of losses identified by referral sources could be said to be influenced by the questions asked, the selection of which losses to include in the referral, and by the often restricted notion of what constitutes a loss.

Group Therapy Referral Reviewed

Total Number of "Loss and Recovery" Group Therapy Referrals Reviewed = 380

Deaths = 84
death of parent 30
death of son by suicide 2
relational suicides 9
pregnancy losses (one abortion) 7
death of daughter (murdered) 1
death of son (shot) 1
death of spouse 4
death of brother 6
death of multiple siblings within short time 2
multiple deaths within last 6 months 1
death of aunt 2
death of girlfriend's child 1
death of neighbor 1
death of sister-in-law 1

death of grandparent 6
death of friend
death of son
suicide of husband
sister's death by suicide
mother's death by suicide
death of therapist 2
therapist suicide 1
death of caretaker 1
anniversary of mother's death due to AIDS

Separations/Relationships = 47
breakups
conflicts

Loss of Custody of Children = 44
loss of custody
potential loss of custody

Numerous Losses = 41
multiple losses over brief time
multiple losses over longer time

Loss of Job = 39
problems holding a job
unemployment
loss of business
retirement

Divorce = 29
divorce
impending divorce

Personal Health Issues = 27
own health losses 2
severe heart problems 1
back injury 1
mastectomy 1
Huntington's disease 1
osteoarthritis 1

deteriorating physical condition 1
dealing with pain 2
AIDS—limited life expectancy 2
loss of sexual potency 2
own health—mental illness 2
loss of self-care
chronic mental illness
multiple hospitalizations 3
loss of potential to have future children 2
loss of independence 3
loss of lifestyle

Other Losses Relating to Relationships = 27
relationship problems 4
loss of placement home with family
loss of community acceptance
abandonment by parent 1
relational affairs 3
no contact with children
empty nest 6
family estrangement due to long-term psychiatric dysfunction
loss of familial support
loss of means of support
loss of self-confidence
rejection of family due to mental illness 1
parent has Alzheimer's/dementia and does not recognize
   person 2
placement of significant other in nursing home
possible loss of therapist
termination with primary care physician

Loss of Housing = 21
loss of housing
homeless
loss of independent living in apartment

Loss of Health of Significant Others = 6
parental health
serious illness of friend

terminal illnesses of girlfriend, mother, husband 3
concern for aging aunt

Loss of Pets = 5
death of pets

Other Significant Losses = 10
property loss 2
numerous traumas 1
loss of church 2
motor vehicle accident 1
rape 1
loss of respect re racial bigotry
loss of license
loss of insurance

Notice that although death is the primary reason for referral, it represents only 22 percent of the referrals. This is not to say that the grief over the death of a significant person is not important, rather out of 380 referrals for complicated grieving it is often one of many reasons for referral for therapy.

Types of Losses That Grieving People Identify As Important

The rule of thumb in bereavement counseling is that every incident identified as a loss is significant to the individual. Only as time passes can one tell which losses will be considered of greater or less significance in one's life. A good example of this principle is seen in the list of losses that patients in a psychiatric facility list as the loss that is most important at any given time. Although they might list losses cited in the previous review sample, they often rate the following as significant and spend just as much time processing these losses.

Losses Related to Mental Illness and Psychiatric Hospitalization

> Freedom
> Dignity
> Respect

Restricted movement
Choice of housing
Choice of relationships
Legal constraints
Guardians
Labeling
Independence
Sociable connections
Individualized treatment
Hope
Loss of essence of self
Faith/beliefs
Treatment
Discharge/"placement"
Knowledge
Privacy
Being my own person

Losses Related to Aging and Residence in a Nursing Home

Elders in a nursing home have their own list of losses and their own grief responses that may be addressed and may also be overlooked. Elders, however, are usually able to name many of these losses quite clearly. Typical losses addressed by nursing home residents include:

Inability to do what I was able to do
Lack of family visits
Loss of parents and death of many peers and siblings
Loss of ability to eat what they want when they want
Lack of personal things
Loss of interests and hobbies
Loss of control of finances
Loss of home
Loss of ability to express strong positive or negative feelings
Loss of ability to dance
Loss of style and fashion
Loss of intimacy
Loss of shaving oneself
Loss of bathing or going to the bathroom as desired

Loss of contact with young people
Loss of ability to contribute

Losses Related to Aging and Declining Health

In another sample, people who are growing older experienced losses that are a part of aging and in many cases part of their declining health. These losses are often experienced even when one remains in his or her own house or apartment.

Lack of privacy
Lack of control
Fear of loss of driving license/car
Loss of memory, eyesight, hearing, mobility
Changes of health care providers/doctor
Loss of role as parent
Loss of control regarding who enters one's home
Loss of appearance—who is this old person
Loss of time
Losses listed previously related to aging

Other losses important to consider ahead of time are those that come from developmental stages (losses that affect infants, children, adolescents, young adults, midlife changes, growing old) and losses resulting from identity issues related to gender, race, faith, sexual identity and preference, and culture. Losses related to acute and chronic illness, organic challenges, and changes in functioning are also important and may make grief complicated.

Sharing Responsibility for Care

Caring for dependent older family members can cause unexpected changes and grief responses even when handled constructively. This was true for Dee who was in her new job less than a year when her mother had a stroke that left her right side paralyzed. Dee's life was going well. She had been promoted at work and was in the midst of moving into her own office when she received news about her mother's stroke. In the midst of packing, Dee stopped long enough to tell her story.

The stroke left her mother greatly weakened and unable to say many words. She was an independent woman who was now highly frustrated and in need of much help. So, Dee resigned her job and was leaving in one week to move back to her childhood home to help with nursing care.

All this Dee shared in a somewhat philosophical manner. She had not expected this, she said. But here she was, part of the sandwich generation. She had just sent her children off to college and now, for the foreseeable future, which could be a very long time, she would be taking care of her mother.

Numerous losses had occurred in Dee's family over the past ten years and she listed them all. Her sister had been taking care of their mother. But Ginny had done more than her share, Dee insisted, and to top it all off, Ginny's husband had been killed last year. "As a matter of fact," Dee said, " I feel I need to do my share."

THE UNIVERSAL, NORMAL GRIEVING PROCESS

Grief As Journey

Grief has frequently been described as a journey. In using this combination of symbol and imagery the person experiencing loss is imagined as going from one place to another and then returning or ending up someplace else. Journeys can be unexpected, spontaneous, desired and undesired, prepared for and catch us unprepared. In this sense, journey is a wonderful image for the grief experience because it presents the basic healing context for grief's story to be told.

Often the journey of grief is depicted as a descent into a valley, the bottom of the valley being the depth of sorrow. This valley is not the peaceful valley of rest but one that comes as a result of tumbling down a deep emotional and spiritual incline and landing on a more troubled plateau for a time before ascending. We all understand journeys and we know that they involve stepping out from our everyday life at least for the time being.

Imagine if you will the grief experience of the nursery rhyme characters, Jack and Jill. Jack and Jill go up the hill to fetch a pail of water. There they are on an ordinary day doing what they need to do. On this journey they will get water to drink, or to do the laundry, or to play with, or just to water the flowers. But, alas, Jack has an accident and tumbles down the hill. Consequently he hurts his head and if that weren't challenging enough, Jill comes tumbling after! Presumably they are both a bit scraped up and X rays may show that Jack needs to be treated for a concussion, and if the injury is truly serious he may have some brain damage. At the very least this is literally an upsetting experience!

There they sit having lost the water and the direction and control of their day and destiny. One or both of them may have hospitalization and other losses coming in the immediate future. In the story, and in their grief, they find themselves in a valley that is filled with a jumble of feelings and thoughts as well as other things—such as ambulances, medical people, family at home worrying about them, and to top it all off, they're probably covered with spilled water.

In my childhood memory, this is the end of this nursery tale. There is life (hills to climb, quests to undertake, tasks to do) and then there is loss and grief and problems to solve. This is true pathos.

This grief story ends with the unstated truth that Jack and Jill will surely have to get up, get help, and decide how they will proceed in life. After treatment, they may decide to get water from easier hills, they may use sturdier shoes as foundation for journeys that can prove difficult, and they may let the adults carry heavy things such as pails of water. Many changes could be made as they recover from this unfortunate episode that ended so terribly.

Thus it is with the journey of life and the journey through the land or valley of grief. These types of journey symbols, images, analogies, and metaphors are all strong tools for understanding grief. When these tools are appropriately used they stand on their own with the power to create empathy, movement, change, and healing. No one ever needs to actually say to a little child who has just heard Jack and Jill, "Now remember dear, there are challenges in life, and you will be faced with loss and grief from which you will need to figure out how to recover."

Grief As Process

Grief is also described dynamically in terms of process, tasks, phases, and stages. This view is closely related to the journey imagery but more acceptable to clinical assessment and inquiry. The process begins with an understanding of the internal responses to loss and of the interpersonal and behavior effects. Normal grieving is said to occur when one engages in the grieving process by working through various stages/phases and tasks. When all, or almost all, of the identified grief work is completed the person is said to have recovered from the loss.

Processes, like journeys, have beginnings, middles, and endings even though they may be difficult to discover and may involve circular and spiral-type return to earlier stages and tasks prior to completing the process. In fact, the term process is helpful because it is paradoxically doable and yet never completely done.

Process then, has the advantage of adding detail to journey. Here are the components of energy, direction, and at the same time limitless happening without concern for chronology or beginnings and endings. In this sense the way one journeys is just as important as the journey. The way one grieves is just as important as the event of grieving.

Grief Is Both Process and Journey

In this book we will be using both process and journey to describe grief. These two companionable descriptions are found in the journey of grief images presented in Figure 1.1. The journey of grief is represented pictorially through the valley image. The process of grief is described through the use of labels, or process markers, along the way.

A LOSS AND RECOVERY MODEL OF GRIEF

In the model of grief that follows, the process of grief is described through the use of these process markers. For the sake of a structural view of grief, these markers, when described in this context and sequence, constitute the universal grief response, or six stages of grief. Throughout the book the combination of grief story (journey) and grief process (stages) has proven helpful in the most severe forms of complicated and dysfunctional grieving.

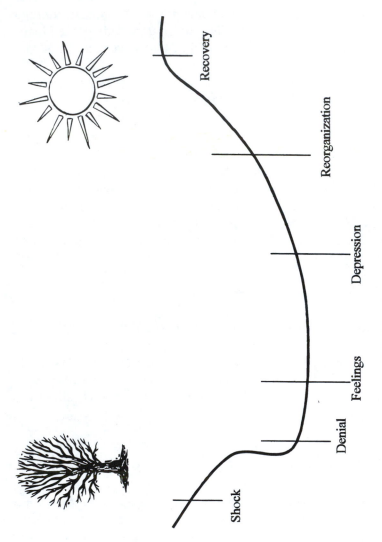

FIGURE 1.1. The Journey of Grief

Shock

Denial

Feelings

Depression

Reorganization

Recovery

The Six Stages of Grief

There are numerous subtle variations available when selecting a stage model of grief. Most variations involve the naming of individual stages or subcomponents of a stage. Since most are sound, any one of these models can be used. However, in clinical practice, it is important to choose a simple model that is fairly jargon free and easily described and remembered by persons who are grieving and by those who help them. The following model fits both of these needs. It is practical, clinically useful, based on solid theory and research, and has been applied with positive outcomes.

This model has six stages of grief that follow a significant loss (see also Appendix A). These stages are based on the assumption of

Significant attachment
Followed by loss

The grieving stages consequent to a significant loss include:

> Stage 1: Shock and numbness
> Stage 2: Denial
> Stage 3: Feelings
> Stage 4: Depression
> Stage 5: Reorganization
> Stage 6: Recovery

Stage 1: Shock and Numbness

Shock is a physiological response to loss. It occurs automatically. Thus it is a biological response built into the human being at birth. The shock response commonly consists of a slackening of the jaw, a widening and freezing of focus in the eyes, and a brief stilling of the body. During this time there are no feelings and no thoughts. In fact, the stilling of feelings and thoughts happens to allow the person experiencing the loss to put all his or her energy into seeing what is happening or hearing what is being said.

As a first alarm, shock and the resulting numbness can last for less than a second and remain for a few minutes or a few hours. Sometimes, when the loss is extremely tragic, painful, or unfathomable, a person can go in and out of a modified phase of being in shock for days or even a week or more. After this relatively brief experience of taking in the fact of a loss the person does not usually return to the initial shock stage during the rest of the grieving process. Although certain aspects and circumstances around a loss can bring smaller experiences of shock, the overall experiences of shock and numbness is time limited.

Stage 2: Denial

The first thoughts after learning of a loss are also somewhat predictable and automatic. The purpose of these thoughts is to protect the newly grieving person from the impact of the loss. In a sense, the person takes momentary flight from the loss. This modulation of feelings and thoughts is essential to defend the self from that which can otherwise threaten to be overwhelming. When working with grieving persons, the image of wrapping a warm coat around oneself works as a description of the positive function of denial and its role in the grief process.

Most of the early denial responses are easily identified. A person often declares some version of the following:

> "No way. This can't be happening."
> "I can't believe it."
> "But I just saw him."

More subtle forms of denial are often found intermittently throughout the grieving process. In fact, it is common for some aspect of denial to occur during each of the consequent stages. A person may deny that he or she feels angry or ashamed. A person may deny that she has moments of intense sadness. A person may deny that he is spending time trying to sort out the relationship. In these latter stages, the function of denial remains the same, to protect the person and to gain time and temporary distance. The actual denial of the fact of the loss varies however from loss to loss and person to person and may be more possible over subtler or less tangible losses.

Stage 3: Feelings

Feelings begin to develop soon after the loss is recognized. Usually feelings are expressed one at a time with one feeling likely to be dominant. During the moments of shock and denial any developing feelings are likely to be subservient to the need to process what happened and to create some protective distance from the event and its impact.

For many people, first feelings are expressed in anger or a form of anger. For some the form of anger is expressed in aspects of blaming, efforts to establish control, or discovering what happened. It is important to remember that what appears to be a thought can really be less of a container of content than it is an expression of feeling. For example, "What the heck happened?" when asked at an early stage may serve the purpose of gathering facts about a loss. It may also have the sole purpose of expressing denial. Or the same response may have the function of expressing anger in an acceptable manner.

As a rule, people who tend to get angry quickly will feel anger as a first response. It helps to think of those whose normal feeling responses tend to fall in the mad (anger) or the sad (bad) categories. It is likely that an individual response will at first relate to his or her preferred feeling response. Often feelings of guilt and fear may underlie feelings of frustration, anger, and even sadness and regret. Frequently feelings of relief are also felt although this may be the most difficult feeling to identify and express. Underlying sadness may include many feelings including despair and disappointment.

The feeling stage of grief is often extensive both in time and in intensity. For feelings to become a constructive part of grief, as many feelings as possible need to be identified and somehow expressed. All feelings expressed are real and should be treated as such. During the next stage the person will have the information and the strength to decide how his or her feelings relate to the loss as a whole. At this point the grief work is to let oneself have feelings and to do so safely.

Stage 4: Depression

When the predominant feeling settles into a sense of sadness or sorrow the depression stage is beginning to occur. However, this stage cannot be constructively entered until other feelings have been explored. Early feelings of sadness have the function of self-expression. However, in the depressive stage sadness is not so much of a protest as it is a lingering missing of the person/relationship or loss that is of significance to the grieving person.

Grief depression is described as a sorrowing grief rather than a clinical grief. It is not major depression. Grief depression is an active and working stage whose purpose is to accomplish three things. These three tasks are usually accomplished sequentially. They may take moments, months, or years to fully complete. However, one can move on to reorganization and partially back into a depression task while remaining in a normal grieving process.

The functions of grief depression are to help the person:

- Review
  - To feel sadness
  - To process feelings
  - To process thoughts
  - To sift and sort through the relationship
- Envision
  - To recognize the loss and its significance
  - To increase awareness of the impact of the loss
  - To notice changes caused by the loss
- Decide
  - To move on

During the review function of depression the person reflects on his or her various feelings and thoughts that have surrounded the loss. This review process is energized by a natural human tendency to think about and sort through relationships. The good is remembered. The challenging is identified. In some cases this can be summed up as looking at the "good, the bad, and the ugly," parts of the relationship. During the review process the thinking or reflective function seems to balance the feeling or sorrow function so that both can occur as long as needed. Toward the end of the review process there is a summing up of the relationship and a settling in to an internal narrative about the relationship. Summation phrases sound like the following:

> "She tried to control every aspect of our life but she really did care and provide for us."
> "He was a mean drunk and made my mother's life miserable but he didn't deserve to die in so much pain."

"I really hated that job. I had trouble doing it. I liked some of the people but that job really wasn't the best job for me."
"She lived a long and full life. She was a good person. I will miss her. Thank goodness she left me with a positive view of life."

Once the relationship has been reviewed the person is able to look briefly into the future and envision possible changes that will occur as a result of the loss. During this time old feelings and even new ones may arise. When glimpsing the future it is normal for a person to briefly go back to the feelings stage but not usually for a long period unless unexpected information (thoughts, feelings, facts) is introduced. Usually the review process, when concluded, comes to the rescue as a way to view what happened and a way to view the impact the loss may have on the future.

Changes that are anticipated are not often extensively thought out at this point. Those that have the most imminent impact are noted. More subtle attention to changes may take some time to become evident. It is not uncommon for some review and envisioning to happen years after a loss. Usually, however, this latter review and envisioning does not have the intensity and pervasiveness of the sadness one felt when first experiencing depression.

The decision to move on is internal and unique to each individual. It is often possible for an individual to identify the internal words they said to themselves, or the time and context of their decision to say good-bye and/or to turn to the future. People who have a prominent thinking function may remember thinking:

> "I've got to move on."
> "I've got to get back to my life."
> "I've got to face tomorrow."

Those who have a prominent feeling function may remember feeling a sense of moving on:

> "I just sensed that it was time."
> "I felt I needed to move."
> "I felt I had cried a river and there were no more tears."

Stage 5: Reorganization

Reorganization is the learning or skill phase of recovery that focuses on changes in one's life as a result of loss. Sometimes a person is aware from the beginning that changes will occur as a result of the loss. Often this awareness of change contributes to the range of feelings and the nature of the depressive sorting that needs to happen. However, it is important to remember that changes can be needed internally as well as externally. Often reorganization involves a combination of the two.

As one woman stated, "When the children were growing up I took care of them. I took care of my husband who did everything by a very strict timetable. He was the one in charge of where we went and what we did. I had no idea how to write a check or even where the account was located. When my husband died I had no idea how to live my days. I had never lived on my own. Even though I didn't get married until later in life, even when I was a young adult I lived at home with my parents. I hate being at home. Now that I don't get around as well; I don't even get out much. How am I supposed to live my life? I could have many more years to live."

All change involves learning. That is what makes change so difficult. While some kinds of learning are fun, learning after a loss is seldom easy in the beginning. It involves concentration, motivation, resources, and energy.

In addition to the obvious changes following a loss there are so many unanticipated changes. The greater the loss the more involved the change. The more involved the change, the more feelings arise that can tend to keep grief acutely present in a person's life. Also, the less the change is wanted or valued, the more difficult the process of reorganization can become.

Finally, the changes that follow a loss may simply be small adjustments. A person's adaptability, in general, can be a strong factor in how well and how long reorganization takes. Plus, a personal preference for action, or contemplation, may make the depression stage more suited to contemplation and the reorganization stage more suited to the action.

Stage 6: Recovery

Making new attachments and investing more energy in ongoing relationships is the task that needs to be completed during the last stage of grief. This investment includes people, objects, interests, and a life that is of value. It must be noted, however, that normal grieving has the objective of returning the person to everyday living. When an individual had difficulty living before a specific loss there may be a need for looking at unresolved grief from other losses or other factors that need to be assessed.

Brad was a hard worker all his life. He was a serious person who never really had much of a sense of humor. He did his job and supported his family. He was quiet and kept social events to a bare minimum. One wouldn't know by looking at him whether he was happy or unhappy. He lived each day pretty much the same way. When Brad's mother died he began to look as though he didn't care about how he dressed or even if he got to work on time. He never said anything. He got by. This went on for almost a year. Then, on the anniversary of his mother's death he took some flowers to her grave. The next day he pulled out his old sweater, shaved himself and got to work on time. After that he never missed a day's work. Everyone who knew him thought he was back to normal. Still, they never could tell whether he was happy or not happy.

IS THE GRIEF PROCESS THE SAME FOR EVERYONE?

The answer to this question is yes and no. That is the tension between theory that is based on reality and reality itself. Theory describes general reality for a given group, in this case human beings who are experiencing grief. From the vantage point of theory, normal grief is a fairly universal experience that most people have throughout their life. This means that most people go through the six stages mentioned above in somewhat similar order. Since this has been demonstrated anecdotally and through research, we can also safely say that grief is natural and somewhat predictable. We can also say that everyone shares the dynamic that grief is at the same time unique to each person. We can also say that grief takes time and that the time needed to recover from grief varies. So, the grief process that we all share is a natural process that each individual goes through in his or her own way and at his or her own speed. This part is the same for everyone. So grief is natural, unique, and varied.

Grief Is Natural

Grief is a part of life, therefore it is part of our nature and is natural. Since grief is part of the essence of who we are, most of us are able to experience loss and recovery without professional intervention even though there may be intense pain and turmoil during the grief experience.

The Grief Process Is Unique to Each Individual

While normal grieving has its identifiable responses and stages, it is nevertheless unique to each person. The ways people express their denial of loss and any other part of the grieving process vary. Feelings come in differing ways with varying intensities. One person sorts through clothing and objects when depressed while another person sits in a chair for days on end and just thinks about the loss. Some people get angry quickly and others get depressed while avoiding anger. Another person begins to reorganize after a loss by reading and preparing to learn new things, while still another just dives right in and tries one thing after the next. Even though there are differences in the content of each stage, a good rule of thumb in grief work is to affirm the commonality of grief (which is often relieving to an individual) and at the same time point to the uniqueness of each person's grief journey (which is freeing).

Timing for Recovery from Grief Varies

It takes time to grieve. Therefore it takes time to recover. This is one of the few universal rules about grief. However, it is one of the most challenged principles of grieving and tends to lead to some of the most challenging complications and dysfunctional responses. This is because our culture, our society, and our environmental context is a strong shaper of process. In the case of a universal or common experience, such as loss, each culture and family has had ample time to solidify explicit and implicit norms for the process and the time that "should" be allotted to it.

The workplace may give an employee three to four days to grieve. Some places give no paid time. After a precise time the person is expected to be back to work. To make matters worse, most losses are not considered significant enough to warrant time off.

Some losses are processed in a few weeks. Such may be the case when the eighty-year-old cousin that one has not seen in ten years dies peacefully in her sleep. Some losses may take several years. Such may be true of the loss of a parent who had a very painful disease and is now out of pain and believed to be in a better place of peace and companionship. Some losses may take ten years to grieve. Such may be true of a divorce that was very painful and undesired and is complicated by custody issues and financial challenges.

The question of the time it takes to grieve and the importance of taking time is illustrated in the case of a fiftyish woman who called to talk. It was the anniversary of her father's death and she was having a difficult time. After listening to her talk for a while I wondered how long ago her father had died. I was quite convinced that the death had been fairly recent. I guessed that it had been within the past three years. To my amazement, it had been thirty years, but it seemed like yesterday to this woman. Still, her grief sounded fresh and raw and she knew that she still hadn't recovered.

GRIEF TRAJECTORIES AND VARIATIONS WITHIN THE NORMAL GRIEF RESPONSE

The journey of grief as described in the earlier part of this chapter, and pictured in Figure 1.1, is just one picture of normal grief. It shows one path through the stages of grief, one trajectory. Other variations are possible. All of these variations could be normal and represent uncomplicated grieving. None of these variations necessarily implies differences in the depth of grieving or pain experienced.

Types of Grief Journeys

Straightforward and Sequential

This is the journey as pictured in Figure 1.1. In this grieving process grief moves from stage 1 to stage 2 and so on through stage 6.

Circular

In this experience of grieving, one may go back and forth between stages. This back-and-forth movement picks up unfinished processing in previous stages. Eventually, however, the person recovers.

Longer at One Stage Than Another

It is also common for a person to stay in one stage much longer than other stages. The stages that commonly take longer are denial, feelings, depression, and reorganization. However, some people say that the feeling stage and the sadness during depression are the most difficult to get through. This is probably due to the pain during these stages and the awareness of that pain. Those in denial may be there for a long time, or in certain ways, but not be aware of it.

Intermittent/Over a Longer Time

In the grieving experience a person may go through one or more of the stages and then stop grieving for a period of time. Later on, other stages may become prominent or other levels of grieving may become important. Their grieving is not constant but the work does eventually get done and the person's life does go on while the grieving process is still occurring.

Lifelong Missing of Lost Object/Person/Dream

It may be said that a lifelong missing of a significant person, dreams, or object should be termed complicated or dysfunctional grieving. However, this grief experience may be normal. It may be true for parents who have lost children. It may be true for elders who have lost spouses and live another ten or twenty years. A lifelong missing of a person, object, or dream may occur even though the person goes through the stages of grief and goes on with life. To determine whether grief is normal, complicated, or dysfunctional more complete assessments need to be made.

Lifelong Unacceptable Loss

Some losses are so traumatic, so horrific, so far reaching in consequences and implication for the human condition, in general, that they remain intact on the human heart and mind as an unrecoverable grief that one lives with and even transcends in functional and creative ways. The Holocaust and other genocides are forever unacceptable. The assassinations of crucial and beloved leaders are forever unacceptable. Slavery and servitude based on race, culture, religion, and gender are forever unacceptable. The normal trajectory for grief in these cases is to find ways to witness and to prevent future generations from these experiences.

ASSESSMENT OF A PERSON'S CURRENT GRIEVING PROCESS

The assessment of whether or not an individual is grieving in a normal way includes rating or describing a person's ability to do the following:

- Identify the loss or losses experienced
- Identify the grieving stage(s) experienced
- Identify where one is in the grieving process
- State how the individual knew that he or she was "moving on"
- Talk about the changes one's made in life
- Share what life is like now, including new connections made
- Reflect on the impact of the loss and the grief process given current awareness

During the assessment of an individual's grief process the person helping the grieving individual needs to determine whether the person's grief is normal and what further help might be useful. In order to make this assessment the helper must:

- Listen to the person talk about losses
- Identify grieving stage(s) according to observable criteria
- Identify verbal expressions of loss/grief
- Consider nonverbal clues, if any, and the meaning of these clues

- Consider unresolved issues, if any
- Assess current lifestyle and changes made

MANAGEMENT OF THE NORMAL GRIEVING PROCESS

In general, normal grief does not require much professional intervention unless that is the choice of the individual. Interventions that occur are often time limited and involve working with moderate complications and mildly interfering behaviors. The management of normal grief remains primarily, and almost exclusively, in the hands of the person experiencing grief and the results are usually successful recoveries. When this is the case, management usually includes a selection of appropriate resources including the sharing of one's grief with significant others. Some of these resources are included in the following text.

Self-Management

As stated previously, the grieving person usually handles normal grieving processes, without formal therapy, with brief therapy, and/or with limited use of medication. This does not mean the person undergoes the process alone, rather that there is a degree of confidence and self-esteem already in place and an internal willingness to go through the process and to set it up so it meets specific needs.

Supportive People, Relationships, and Beliefs

Normal grieving processes can involve numerous supportive connections from family, from first line social/spiritual contacts in the community, or specialized support groups. In fact, it is now common for people to attend support groups in their community. These groups help the person get through the stages and experiences of grief.

Popular Literature

Numerous books and other literature are available for the grieving person who is experiencing normal grief. These materials are found in public places such as libraries, newsstands, bookstores, hospitals, and churches. Most of these materials are well written and solidly based. Usually the person seeks these resources out and/or responds well to suggestions.

Time

Many persons who have experienced grief feel that time was a healing factor for them. With or without conscious help from supportive people or other resources, many people believe that time contributes to recovery. In most cases the reference to time is a popular way to describe the grieving process. Those who have never heard about the stages of grief still know that it took time for them to recover.

Cultural Values, Rituals, and Ceremonies

Cultural values, rituals, and ceremonies continue to help persons process their grief in normal and acceptable ways. In a pluralistic world, there are now many new ways to grieve. This variety can be a resource to grieving persons. It contains the grief and legitimizes it at the same time.

Talk

The primary treatment for grief is talk. A grieving person is best helped by having other persons listen to his or her experiences of loss. As one person put it, "I have a right to cry. I have a right to have these feelings." Talking is a primary way for grief to be expressed. However, it is not the only way. In some cases, a person's use of words needs to be brief and to the point. At other times, talking needs to continue for some time. Many people need to tell their story again and again. All this can be quite normal.

SUMMARY

In the effort to learn more about helping people manage complicated grieving, the review of normal and uncomplicated grief is essential. The stage theory of grief presented here will remain the basis for understanding how complications develop and changes that need to occur in the course of recovery from loss. The truth is one can never go far from the basic grief responses and processes when working with responses that are extremely challenging. Even the most complicated responses are helped by the juxtaposition of how grief normally progresses.

Chapter 2

When Grief Becomes Complicated

> Like a cut on your hand, the crisis or grief wound will gradually heal over time, unless it is infected. But in our death-denying culture of massive loneliness, many people experience some degree of infection when they are so wounded. The infection may retard or totally block the healing process.

> Clinebell, 1992, pp. 224-225

While loss tends to be resolved through natural healing processes, this is not always true. Sometimes, the grieving process that follows significant loss can become quite troublesome and problematic. Furthermore, troublesome and problematic grief responses may lead to even more extensive complications. In fact, it is sometimes surprising how rapidly grief can become complicated.

This awareness of the potential for grief to become complicated is a crucial step in helping people through the grief process. Once one is aware of the potential for grief to become complicated, one is in a position of understanding the importance of resources and the need for effective and timely interventions. The awareness of the potential for complications to arise within any grieving process serves as a reminder to all of us of the fragility of life and the complexity of our experiences of connection and disconnection.

Unfortunately, awareness can also lead to the development of fears and anxiety about the impact of loss in general. When this happens, professionals and helpers may experience being caught up in a parallel process of complicated grief about grieving! Such is often the situation with people who are new, inexperienced, or have been in the field so long that their objectivity has become somewhat distorted.

Yet in a creative sense, the understanding of complications that can and do occur within the grief process, can lead one to a more compassionate alertness and to proactive responses. When this is the case, one develops a more genuinely supportive stance and is moved to become more skilled in the provision of treatment. In such instances, awareness of complications can lead to an emphasis on continued development of capacity and ability to meet more caring and therapeutic needs of grieving individuals.

In this chapter, complicated grief is explored by looking at the root causes of complications, the risk factors that can become predictors of complicated grief, and the complications that arise during specific stages of grief. In addition, examples of complicated grieving are presented to increase insight and understanding of experiences of complicated grief. However, it is important to keep in mind that the potential for complications does not mean that complications will definitely occur even when some, or many, of these factors are present.

In fact, predicting complicated grief responses is somewhat like umpiring a football game. During the game it is the referee's job to pay attention to gains that are made, losses, and fouls committed during the course of play. All are announced immediately after they occur. The gains lead to progress and maybe new points on the board. However, when a foul is observed, a red flag is thrown to the ground. The game is stopped and the referees take a closer look at what seems to have gone wrong. A similar situation occurs when complications arise during an otherwise normal grieving process.

In the midst of normal grieving there are times when a red flag may seem to be metaphorically thrown to the ground as a note of caution. This flag, when it appears, suggests that grief may be going somewhat "afoul" of its normally intended function and process. The question then arises as to what has gone wrong or become complicated about the process. Training and experience in grief care and counseling increases the professional ability to recognize what might be becoming complicated. In fact, grieving individuals should also be taught to pay attention to their own processes and to grow in their ability indicate where and when they may need help.

In the following vignette, a young woman actually throws out her own flag to indicate she is in the midst of complicated grieving. She does so by boldly calling grief itself into question. This she does with pain, anger, and a bit of naiveté. Unfortunately, even though she knows that her grief is not working, she doesn't yet know that she can be helped. Yet, she sends up a flag that is designed to get help in its own dramatic way.

STORIES OF COMPLICATED GRIEF

A young woman sits on the couch with one foot resting on the coffee table. Her head rests on her arm and her long hair hides most of her face. She has experienced several deaths in her family over the past years and as she speaks she is aware of several more relatives and acquaintances who are dying. She believes that those who have already died are better off in heaven. When asked about her grieving process she declares with a hint of anger. "It's no use grieving. What difference does it make?" The rest of her peers remain silent. She says no more. When the leader mentions that grieving happens to all of us even though it happens in different ways with different people, the young woman glares at the leader and says, "Who are you anyway?" and leaves the room.

Some would say she is in denial and they would be right. Some would say she is filled with a variety of natural emotions that are descriptive of that grieving stage. They, too, would be right. A further possibility would be to assess that this young woman is in the depressive-sadness phase of grieving and is stuck in that sorting process. This makes sense. However, no one would say that she is in the reorganization phase of grief. That is why she has been referred to this loss and recovery group. Finally, all of us would probably be correct if we assumed that this young woman might be headed for a complicated grieving process or currently stuck in the midst of one.

To be honest, given just the contact previously noted, it is not possible to know this young woman's grief, loss history, or her story. But it is possible to know some of the meaning she currently makes of it. It is also possible to hypothesize that this woman has a story that is in need of telling, and of being heard!

We already know that her story involves many losses. We can assume that her grief has become overwhelming and has been unproductive. It is of no use! In other words, her grieving process hasn't made things right. She has not recovered.

We can understand her wish. She is not alone in wanting grief to make things right. She is not alone in wanting her life to be right. She is also not alone in having a life story that begins with loss. We can understand these feelings. But, where we differ is that counselors and caregivers know that grief can be healing. It can be helped to be more productive. It can work! Even so, this young woman is entitled to her own experience. So we accept that experience and recognize that she is trying to make meaning out of her life the best way she can.

This is true for all of us. Each of us tries to find meaning the best way we can. For this reason each of us has a story with its own beginning. Many of our stories begin with experiences of joy and celebration. Other stories begin with experiences of grief and loss.

Personal stories of grief and loss often begin with the phrase, "I was all right until . . ." This phrase can be implied or explicit. It can be the theme for individuals, families, organizations, communities and even nations. Frequently, the story that is told in this manner is a story that involves profound loss and grief. Just as frequently, such a story involves experiences of complicated grief.

A young girl's story begins with, "I was all right until that evening in December when a police car came and took my brothers, sister, and me off to a children's home. I was seven years old."

A man's story also has a beginning. "I was all right until I married her. I was middle-aged and everyone else in my family was married. That's when the major depression began."

Another woman's story had a beautiful beginning. "The wedding was beautiful. We set off doves to symbolize how our souls were meant to be together. Then, a couple of months later he says, "I want a divorce. I never loved you."

Everyone has a story. Here are more beginnings for grief and loss stories that begin with the phrase, " I was all right until . . ."

> my mother got Alzheimer's
> the stroke
> the affair
> the neighbors complained
> the cruiser picked me up
> I got hit with the baseball bat
> I saved the boy and got hit myself
> this irregular lump was found in my breast
> I was diagnosed with liver cancer
> I started drinking

they fired me
my father died
I came here

In our minds, and in our memories, we need to have beginnings. We need to find causes for the experiences that happen to us. These beginnings become for us the record of what has caused our life to be the way it was and the way it has become. While we usually have stories of "wasn't it wonderful when . . ." and "wouldn't it be great if . . ." we especially rely on stories that express our grief experiences and our most painful moments of loss. So we begin our grief stories with "I was all right until . . ." This is how we mark time. This is how we make meaning. These stories contain the seminal points that have changed our lives forever.

As one woman stated in the midst of a grief therapy group, "If I don't blame myself, then how do I make sense out of all that happened? How do I find out what all this means?" In the telling of her grief story, she begins with, "It was all my fault. I brought this on myself. I was all right until I stopped listening. I behaved like a brat. I was mean. I deserve all this." Her tears overflowed. For months her grief story remained the same and she stood by it with fierce defensiveness. Every effort to wonder about the story or to edit any portion of it would only go so far when she would run back to the safety of the earlier edition. Only this story made sense to her. The other story was so horrible she could not face it. The other story, that she had developed a severe case of depression that had to do with her brain, was unacceptable. In her mind's eye and memory bank her environment and actions were the causes of loss and relentless grief and dysfunction. She could not accept that both were true and that there was still more truth to be found in the functioning of those around her before and after she became depressed.

As a rule of thumb, people who have had significant losses tell stories of loss, of grief, and of their attempts to recover. In the telling of their stories, they make their own interpretations as to how their grief experience has affected their life. There is much drama and passion in the story even if the feelings are suppressed.

Those who have recovered tell all this in a straightforward way. There is richness to their recovery story. The person adds what she or he knows or has learned along the way. She or he is able to share process, challenges, and accomplishments. This story is alive. It continues to bring insight as a result of being shared one more time. It goes into the future.

For those who are still grieving, or whose grief is complicated, the story includes hidden and explicit negative feelings—anger, guilt and/or sadness, and sometimes intense blaming. There may be a continued sense of numbness, denial, or avoidance. Those whose grief has become complicated over time may tell a story that is somewhat flat and rigid. They don't necessarily know that their story is just a hypothesis. So they are not open to the development of new editions that will come as they continue to work productively through their grief. Thus their grief story is less active and changing than those whose grief is normal. In normal grief, the experience, and therefore the story, is a work in progress that changes over time. Even when the person is in denial, or the grips of strong feelings, he or she is tentatively open to the possibility that his or her grief will change in the future. But, for those whose grief is complicated, one senses, upon hearing their story, that they are stuck in their story and that it is running them. Yet, it is this grief story, told the way a person needs to tell it, that the professional helper will want to hear again and again for it carries within it the seeds of a more authentic story that will someday, hopefully, be transformed in recovery.

IS GRIEF BECOMING MORE COMPLEX?

One day a colleague and I took a break after coleading two loss and recovery groups in a psychiatric in-patient setting. The groups had been difficult, filled with anger, pain, and deep sorrow. Many of the losses were horrendously traumatic. The grief responses included an ongoing list of self-harming behaviors, dysfunctional relationships, and mental, emotional, and spiritual complications. Back in the office, just before lunch, I turned to my colleague and asked, somewhat rhetorically, "Is grief becoming more complex, or am I just imagining it?" We commiserated with each other convinced that the correct answer was all, none, or some of the above. We were currently in no condition to think clearly. So we talked about what happened in group and about how we felt. This was the way we recovered from the pain that came with compassionate caring and the intense therapeutic work of this day.

It may be that there is no definitive answer to this question at this time. But the question remains a concern for many counselors, clergy, health care providers, and organizations. Needless to say, if this hypothesis is correct, the question is also one that concerns grieving individuals and their loved ones. For if grief is becoming more complicated, there is an increased need for resources to help people recover from these losses and the complications that arise. Yet, an increase in resources would run counter to the current cultural and social custom of decreasing costs through strict monitoring of utilization of services. Maybe the current direction of minimizing the increased complexity of the grieving process seems more manageable, if not realistic.

The following example describes the grief experience of a highly educated and bright family with very good coping skills. Yet the overwhelming complexity of their losses and their grieving bring them to the point of seeking help from a health care provider. Prior to these experiences neither one would have considered the need for professional help to manage grief.

Melissa's Experiences

Melissa sat at her desk quietly eating her lunch. It was two weeks before Easter and the three women eating lunch together were thinking about the upcoming holiday and how they would celebrate it. Hopes and disappointments were shared equally. When Melissa's turn came, she noted that her sister-in-law was having chemo treatment and that if the treatment happened just before Easter they would postpone the celebration for a week. This made sense to her because Marilyn never felt good right after chemo.

One week later, Melissa's husband, Kevin, got a call from another sister. Her teenage daughter had been in a car accident and her condition was critical. Could he come? There was no Easter. Instead, the whole family gathered at the hospital and hoped for signs that the young girl would survive. She did survive, although no one knew if she would be paralyzed from the neck down. Her spinal column was reattached and her jaw operated upon. She remained on a ventilator.

Another week came and went. This time Kevin received a call from his niece. His brother had gone back to work and had had an accident. Could he come? He dropped everything and flew to his brother's side. He helped to hold his brother down while others cared for his leg. This was an especially difficult task as his brother's leg had to be amputated at the knee. But Kevin was there for his brother. He helped to shave him. He stayed by the bed day and night. He angrily, and somewhat helplessly, witnessed the extreme pain that took several days before it could be effectively relieved.

In the middle of that week, Kevin called home. He had been sent by hospital staff for a medical consult for depression and for counseling. Meanwhile, at home, Melissa was having such a difficult emotional time that she, too, went to her doctor who gave her a prescription for an antidepressant. The losses and grief within the extended family continued even into the next year.

Are Complications on the Rise?

According to Piper and colleagues,

> . . . it is frequently reported that substantial proportions of the population experience unresolved grief and clinical complications. Unresolved grief refers to extremes in the intensity or duration of grief symptoms (e.g., prolonged anguish and preoccupation with the loss or the complete absence of reactions to the loss). Clinical complications refer to a variety of associated problems such as anxiety, depression, health-compromising behaviors, and physical morbidity sometimes leading to death. (Piper, McCallum, et al., 2001, p. 526)

Although there may not be sufficient data to indicate whether complications to the normal process of grieving are on the rise, anecdotal evidence can be gathered from clinicians in the field. To begin with, evidence exists of an increased awareness and seeking of treatment. This may be due to changes and complexity in our environmental context and our relationship to it. Thus the following statements are foundations for hypothesizing an increase in complexity and experiences of complicated grief:

There continues to be an increase in awareness of the grieving process in our society. Much has been written about grief in the past three decades. This material is readily available in bookstores, the library, and on the Internet. Furthermore, an increase has occurred in awareness of grief and loss as evidenced by media foci. Bereavement support groups are numerous, advertised, and available in many areas. Even medications for depression and anxiety, common results of intense grieving, are advertised on television and in popular magazines.

This increase in awareness has led to the seeking of treatment. People frequently seek treatment specifically for losses. Often they self-diagnose, rather accurately, that their grief seems to have taken hold of their life in unhelpful ways. Often the person seeking treatment for significant losses and profound grief feels that he or she is not "snapping back" and is greatly concerned. Others seek treatment for situations other than loss and grief and find that grieving affects what they are seeking treatment for or is discovered in the course of treating the initial issue.

The nature and extent of losses may have increased as a result of changing lifestyles, technology, mass terrorism, and a shrinking, interdependent world. We know that change itself can be a stressor. We also know that change, whether wanted or unwanted, brings experiences of gain and loss. Changes that may affect the complexity of grief experiences are somewhat continuous in our postmodern world. Furthermore, we are less able to block the knowledge and effect of these changes than we were in less industrialized times. Change is brought into our homes through television, the Internet, and through the increasing diversity within the communities where we live, work, go to school, and do all the things we do during the course of our lifetime.

In summary, the prevalence of the experience of loss at a personal and social level cannot be accurately determined without increased research. So, too, does the prevalence of complications remain in question. Yet, anecdotal evidence suggests that the prevalence and complexity of complicated grief may indeed be greater than we have previously suspected.

If the hypothesis that complications are on the rise is true, the task of professional caregivers may remain constant, particularly if the person is well trained in working with persons experiencing complicated grief. In these instances, bereaved people, whose losses seem overwhelming and whose responses often become intense and problematic, continue to need skilled and compassionate help in a timely manner. However, the need for persons with advanced training and willingness to do this time consuming work will increase.

A DEFINITION OF COMPLICATED GRIEF

In an endeavor to provide a comprehensive and clinically practical way to conceptualize complicated grief, the following template can be used to assess thoughts, feelings, beliefs, and behaviors that may indicate complicated grief. By establishing this template we can formulate a working definition of complicated grief.

The three common indicators of health and distress are intensity, duration, and prevalence of symptomatic behavior. Symptomatic behavior includes thoughts, feelings, actions, or the absence of any of these three. These indicators represent fluxuations rather than constant states within a person. The assessment or measurement of these states may provide clear data at some times and be more ambiguous at others.

With these indicators in mind, complicated grief can be defined as grief that follows specific loss, or losses, and meets all three of the following criteria:

1. Complicated grief is especially intense or remarkably absent of intensity.
2. Complicated grief is often very long-lasting.
3. Complicated grief is usually so pervasive that it affects much of a person's daily living and can be observed by professionals, significant others, and perhaps the bereaved person.

Any one criterion is not sufficient, in and of itself, to warrant the use of the term complicated. Nor is any one criterion to be applied without careful examination of the grieving process as experienced by the grieving individual. In making an assessment of whether a person is experiencing complicated grief, a cluster of problematic grief responses should be evident. However, complications that may be evident to an observer may not be as evident to the person experiencing grief.

Putting these three indicators together, complicated grief can be defined as follows:

Complicated grief refers to a holistic grief response that is more intense than would be otherwise indicated. Complicated grief lasts longer than typical grief, and at the same time, it pervasively affects the grieving person's daily life (and behaviors) in significant and negative ways.

Identification of Complications

Since the identification of complicated grief is based on the understanding of normal grief responses, it is crucial to compare each grieving experience with the template of normal grieving (see Chapter 1, the six stages of grief). Allowances are then made for the uniqueness of each person. These allowances or variations can only be assessed when one knows a person well. This personalized grief template will take into consideration specific patterns of behavior, thoughts, feelings, and beliefs. Given a personalized template of normal grieving, one can hypothesize possible complications and even identify them more rapidly as they occur.

This being said, it is also possible and worthwhile to formulate a grief template that generically represents complicated grieving. In constructing a complicated grief template one uses the normal grieving stages and pays attention to what typically interferes with successful journeying through each stage. These interferences are called obstacles or complications.

STAGE-SPECIFIC COMPLICATIONS

Although numerous complications can occur during the grieving process, the following complications represent some of those most frequently observed and most commonly problematic. For more information about complications surrounding significant loss, the reader is encouraged to read further in this text, consult Appendix B, "Possible Complications Surrounding Significant Loss," and refer to the bibliography.

Complications During Shock and Denial

Difficulty Processing Occurrence of a Death or Major Loss

It is a rare occasion when an individual is actually unable to process that a death or major loss has occurred, although it can happen.

For example, people with organic problems such as found in the dementias, in Alzheimer's, or in low developmental functioning, may have difficulty processing that a death or major loss has occurred. People who are actively psychotic may also have problems processing the occurrence of a death or major loss. However, individuals with these processing problems can often be surprising in their ability to understand and experience loss. Often the difficulty processing the occurrence of a death or major loss presents itself in difficulty in attachment, problems with current reality in other areas, and in the ongoing need for individualized support and professional interventions.

Occasionally, the difficulty processing the occurrence of a death or major loss may be due to the horrific nature of the death/loss. Certain losses are complicated simply because they are unfathomable. These losses assault normal reasoning and experience.

Other losses take longer to register because of time factors and distance in relationships. These losses are more understandable but still make processing the fact of loss complicated. In Jason's case, he was not used to seeing his father. His father lived on the other coast and was often overseas. It had been many years since he had seen or talked with his father. Although he received an occasional card, he had no current picture or interaction that made his father real to him. When he was told of his father's death he was informed that it had happened a year ago and everything had been taken care of by those who were close to him. This complication of time and distance in relationship made it harder for Jason to process the fact that his father was dead. It did not seem real.

In another situation, it took a woman a long time to understand that her husband had died. During this time she was treated with medications to stabilize her illness that included symptoms that interfered with her processing of reality. When she finally understood that her spouse had died, she was able to ask for a service to be held on her behalf and in memory of her husband. In this case, her illness became an obstacle to normal grieving. The illness was the complication. She did not understand reality when it happened so she could not process the death even when she had witnessed it.

Denial of the Magnitude of the Loss

A frequent complication in the grieving process surrounds the denial of the importance or magnitude of a loss. This kind of minimization may help a person through certain stages during normal grieving. However, the continued minimization of significant losses eventually undermines healthy grieving. Particularly problematic are efforts to avoid feelings and to avoid the review process that functions as a way of sorting through relationships. People who deny the magnitude of their loss often try, prematurely, to move on without doing the grief work essential to recovery. Only careful attention to the person will determine whether denial of the importance of a loss is happening and what purpose that denial is serving.

Inability to Observe Societal Rituals Surrounding Death or Significant Loss

This can be viewed as a cultural, social, and personal complication. This kind of complication often develops when a culture is in denial about the importance of following certain rituals after a significant loss. In America, viewing a loved one's body, having a service, carefully selecting a spot or process for burial or distribution of ashes, have become somewhat optional. This lack of attention to, or provision of ritual, is true in other circumstances involving loss. In cases of separation, divorce, and loss of custody of children, often such turmoil occurs that grief becomes enveloped in violence, meanness, and/or lack of feeling rather than in positive rituals. When dealing with loss of a job, financial catastrophes, and other changes of great magnitude, positive cultural and social rituals are few and far between.

Rituals have a way of assisting a person through the early phases of shock and denial. They also provide a way for sorrow to be publicly expressed. In this sense, positive rituals often facilitate grief before it has the opportunity of becoming displaced, distorted, or repressed. When a person is not offered bereavement choices after a significant loss, complications can occur. This is true of all losses that are substantial and/or significant.

For example, it is a lingering wound to a grieving person when he or she is not informed of a death at the same time as other family members. It is an additional wound when the individual cannot attend a wake, funeral, or graveside service. It makes no difference whether family members, or others, think they are trying to protect the individual. Just the act of omission from important rituals is a wound that almost always complicates matters.

In one group therapy session, all three persons in the group had at least one significant loss in which they were not told about a parent's death until much later. In one case, a young woman declared, "I don't think my mother is dead. I think she is in hiding." When pushed to explain, she said, "Oh, if I stop to make myself think, I know in my heart that she is dead. But my head says she is alive and hiding. I wanted to see her body but my family said no." This complication was a barrier that continued to contribute to intermittent shock and denial for some years after her mother's death.

Complications During the Feeling Stage

Complications that are most problematic during the feeling stage of grief are those responses whose function is to deny feelings, to make the expression of feelings problematic, result in mixed feelings, or strong singular feelings.

Denial of Feelings

Managing grief when it is forbidden to grieve. In some families, members are explicitly or implicitly forbidden to grieve their losses. Frequently this rule applies to large and small losses alike. The complications that arise as a result of this barrier are difficult to manage, let alone overcome. In this case, the denial of grief is part of the status quo and the repercussions for breaking the rule are often isolation, reprimands, and internal guilt. This style of coping often leads to increased depression and anxiety that are frequently kept hidden in an effort to conform to external expectations.

Problems Expressing Feelings

Lack in capacity to access, identify, or express feelings. The problem in accessing, identifying, or expressing feelings may result from a diminished capacity to feel. Most people are capable of having feelings, but not everyone has ready access to feelings. These people find it hard to get in touch with their feelings. They may have become more comfortable sticking to thoughts and actions. This can be problematic because grief is a process that involves both thoughts and feelings.

Others have not learned how to identify their feelings. If feelings cannot be identified, they cannot be brought to consciousness and honored. Thus, they remain potent sources of energy that at times can be displaced inappropriately on other people, objects, and relationships.

In normal grief work, a feeling is experienced, named for what it is, and expressed in some way. So, a person who feels some relief over the death of a loved one who did not suffer may sense some calmness within and identify that calmness as a feeling of relief. He or she may express this relief by saying to a spouse, "I am sad but I am also relieved that he did not have to suffer for a long time." This is productive grief work. However, if individuals feel that they just can't express their feeling adequately or safely, these may be serious complications.

Mixed Feelings

Ambivalent, violent, overpowering, unsanctioned attachments. Many people have mixed feelings about a loss because seldom is just one feeling involved in grieving. But some feelings are too challenging to handle without help. These feelings are potentially destructive because the energy is held inward or expressed inappropriately.

Ambivalent feelings are not, in and of themselves, complicated. In fact they are rather normal. However, intense ambivalence that brings out intense anxiety can be problematic.

Violent feelings are usually indicators of grief complications. Violent feelings that are extremely intense and lead to preoccupation or plans to act on these feelings place the person at high risk. The desire to do violence to self, or others, can create significant safety issues that must be addressed as quickly as possible with the help of skilled professionals.

Overpowering feelings can lead to difficulty in managing grief and managing appropriate daily functioning at the same time. Violent feelings can be so overpowering that the urge to action may be of great concern. Overpowering sadness and anger can lead to a desire to die. Ambivalent feelings can be so debilitating that decisions are not made, daily activities are stalled, and health may be in jeopardy.

Unsanctioned feelings are also sources of complication. This can be true in the case of extremely positive feelings. If one doesn't feel safe disclosing feelings publicly, this can be a possible complication. Such situations can include same-gender relationships, intimate relationships outside of marriage or partnership, and interracial or class distinctions.

Strong Singular Feelings

Large degree of anger, guilt, and feelings caused by emotional secrets. Strong, intense feelings can be problematic if they become a fixation and exclude other feelings so that the relationship is not realistically reviewed. Some of these fixated feelings are negative. It is actually common to discover that some people choose to be angry, guilty, and ashamed for a long time. This is often true for relationships that are dysfunctional and traumatic, and for relationships that were or are secretive. Plus, relationships that are strongly positive may fixate on one feeling, such as love, to the exclusion of other feelings that would be experienced were they allowed to surface.

Complications During the Depression Stage

Sadness or Sorrow That Becomes Pervasive and Remains Intense over an Extended Time

A certain amount of sadness can be quite normal after a loss and can remain for some time. For example, the loss of a child can be felt for a lifetime and not be considered abnormal grief even though the loss of a child often complicates grief. However, the issue of sadness becomes more complicated when one's life becomes fixated on sorrow, when sadness becomes depression, and when sorrow interrupts crucial life activities for more than brief periods. A complication, as a result of extended sadness and sorrow, usually results in the creation and maintenance of obstacles that limit pleasure and other accomplishments and interactions. When life is restricted for a long time, then grief can be considered complicated.

Lack of Ability/Success in Sorting Through/Reviewing a Relationship

During the depressive stage of grief the bereaved person experiences sadness and sorrow. Over time he or she begins to review his or her relationship to the lost person, object, idea, or belief. The purpose of this review is to open up a broader understanding of one's relationship with that which is lost and the development of a realistic and adequate perspective on what that loss means now.

If a person is not able to do a comprehensive review, the results may be a limited understanding of the effects of the loss and the impact it has on one's life. If one is not able to sort through the loss and its effects, then one does not have the freedom or focus to move on toward recovery. Complications in the review process are usually due to conflicted and intense feelings both positive and/or negative. Personal deficiencies due to internal problems may also make it difficult to separate oneself sufficiently to sort through and gain a more comprehensive understanding of the relationship.

Problems Encountered in Deciding to Move On

Most people have an inner sense of when it is time to move on and finish the intense early part of grief work, but some feel unable to do so. Sometimes the fear and avoidance of moving on arises from a concern about forgetting the person, object, or desired idea or belief. Sometimes the fear is based on a concern that moving on will negate the relationship and therefore part of one's self will be lost. At other times the decision to move on is stalled from fear of changes that may lie ahead.

One person stated her problem in this area thusly, "I've been in denial, I've expressed my feelings, but I stay stuck in a mixture of sadness and anger. Why can't I move on?" Another person declared with conviction, "I don't want to accept it. I can't. What if I don't want to recover?"

Complications During the Reorganization Stage

Difficulty Learning New Skills

All change requires learning. Yet learning is not always considered a good thing. In fact, some people just hate to learn new things. They don't feel competent in their capacity to learn. They don't feel they are successful learners due to unfinished grief over previous attempts. Others resent being forced to make changes as the result of a loss that was not their choice. When the degree of change required is great, and significant resistance is encountered to learning new things, the chances of developing complicated and or dysfunctional grieving increase proportionately.

Unwillingness to Make Necessary Changes

Many people do all the grief work right up through sorting out the changes that have to be made, then they stop. They know what needs to be done and choose not to do it, or, they begin to do what needs to be done but do it poorly, often investing the least possible amount of energy. Their heart and determination are not in it. In some cases, a cessation of strong feeling creates a secondary numbness, denial, and lethargy. This unwillingness to make necessary changes can be blatant, subtle, or everywhere in between.

People seldom use the direct approach and verbalize their resistance to change. However, one man did so in a most helpful way. After participating in psychoeducational training about posttraumatic stress he declared rather thoughtfully, "My way of living has served me well in the past. I see no need to change." He could now see the effect of early childhood abuse but he declared that he was just "resistant to change." He could not see that this refusal to make necessary changes would further complicate his grief and cause even more dysfunctional behavior.

Sometimes the unwillingness to make even optional changes may result in complicated responses. Often these optional changes are remembered as "should-have, would-have, and could-have" quandaries that provoke strong feelings of remorse even in the light of unpredictable hindsight. Even roads not traveled can be sources of complication. Interestingly enough, these "Monday morning quarterbacking" quandaries are even expressed as losses:

"If I had a dime for every time I thought of doing that."
"If only I had done what she suggested."
"If only I had listened."
"If only I had followed my heart."
"If I hadn't taken the easy way out."

Thus, during reorganization, the choices made or not made can lead to secondary losses and grief that can complicate current attempts to change. Particularly painful are choices that the person thinks or believes he or she could have done but chose not to do.

Complications During Recovery

Struggles with Ongoing Relationships

Stressors involving ongoing relationships can also complicate grieving. In the best of circumstances, relationships support us during periods of difficult loss as well as when we are in periods of recovery, maintenance, and growth. When the same relationships are not supportive during the early part of stage six, recovery, a recently grieving person may become overwhelmed and return to more acute grieving with the additional loss now added to the earlier one.

At times, ongoing relationships directly interfere with normal grieving. In these situations a more active obstacle is set up, intentionally or otherwise. For example, families have ways of grieving that can be problematic and not conducive to healthy recovery. Plus, individuals within families experience loss differently, so tensions rise as recovery happens in differing ways and at differing speeds. In addition, the changes that seem important to recovery may involve struggles over new roles, expectations, and the introduction or exclusion of some people. These familial and personal factors always influence grieving and are significant in making the recovery period just as complicated as the earlier stages.

Diminished/Impaired Capacity to Love Again

A particularly painful and overwhelming loss can leave an individual drained in capacity and willingness to become attached to others. If this diminishment continues for a significant period and is not sublimated or transformed in other ways, the person may be at risk of never fully recovering. In such cases, it is often necessary to engage in therapy to repair the basic developmental issues of safety, trust, and empathy.

Frequently, professionals finish helping a person through the first five stages of grief only to discover that he or she has not successfully completed the recovery process. Thus, at times a difficulty in reattaching to people and to objects or ideas and beliefs can catch the person and professionals by surprise. This difficulty may be more surprising during the final phase of reorganization or early phase of recovery. At these times it is still important to remember that when there is a diminished capacity to love with equal or greater emotional and spiritual energy, the grief is complicated and additional help is needed.

This impairment in attachment can occur even when the person had the initial ability to attach to and/or love others. At the same time it must be remembered that the issue of impaired ability to attach from infancy is another issue. This impairment more appropriately belongs in a discussion of early childhood development problems, which may cause attachment to be either nonexistent or false. These false attachments may be mimicked, or learned responses, for the purposes of gain rather than genuine attachment. To assess whether a diminished or impaired capacity to love is present, one must know whether that capacity was present prior to the loss (or losses) and then determine its prior quality.

Diminished Faith/Trust in the Benevolence of the World/People

In some instances, a person reorganizes his or her life by determining to live alone and/or to become less attached to persons/objects and ideas that once held pleasure. As is the case with relational impairments, when this occurs it is also a spiritual issue. If this complication continues in the reorganization and recovery stages, a sense of global pessimism can become a way of life. Multiple and traumatic losses can have such an effect. Losses that seem to be unfair, make no rational sense, or result in a life cut down prematurely, can have the lasting complication of leaving a person to conclude that the world, creation, and people are not as benevolent as previously thought.

GENERAL RISK FACTORS

Identification of Risk Factors

In the section above, complications that arise during the process of grieving are categorized according to some of the tasks, or grief work, that must be completed during the various stages of grief. Another way to approach grief complications is to look at general factors that place a person at risk following a loss. These factors should be considered along with the stage-focused approach. So, having reviewed typical complications during the stages of grief, we now turn to the task of categorizing general risk factors and specific categories of people who are at risk for complications.

Four factors are commonly considered when assessing the potential for normal or complicated grief. They have an impact on all grief responses but take on added significance under specific conditions (see also McCall, 1999, pp. 49-53). The conditions listed beneath each factor are particularly problematic.

1. Nature of the relationship
2. Nature of the loss
3. Physical, psychological, sociological, and spiritual condition of the survivor
4. Resources available to the bereaved

Nature of the Relationship

In general, healthy relationships tend to contribute to normal grieving responses. But healthy is a relative term when it comes to relationships. For, in truth, everyone has at least one relationship that is conflicted, less than functional, or even quite dysfunctional. It is unusual to find a person whose relationships, as a whole, are not somewhat ambivalent or conflicted at one time or another. Yet, some highly conflicted and dysfunctional relationships are grieved in a normal way.

So, although the nature of the relationship a person has with the loss must be examined, this alone will not be sufficient to determine whether grief will become complicated. Still, conflict from particularly violent and abusive relationships usually results in increased risk for complications. However, even conflicted relationships must be assessed in conjunction with next three risk factors and cannot stand alone when making a risk assessment.

Nature of the Loss

The nature or essence of a loss significantly influences the grief process. Certain losses tend to place an individual at risk for complications even if one cannot link that factor with certain causality. Some of the losses that tend to make grief complicated include loss of health, freedom, choice for change, multiple losses, betrayals, and stigmatic and shaming losses.

Loss of Health

A change in health is often a complicating factor for grief. When the loss results in the decline of health so that a possibility of long-term, degenerative, or life-threatening illness exists, that loss of health places an individual at risk for complicated grieving. Particularly painful, unpleasant, and behaviorally challenging illnesses are also problematic. So, too, is any unsavory or unfathomable illness. In any of these situations, the person, whose health has changed dramatically, grieves the loss of health and/or by the health changes that happen to people he or she cares about.

Loss of Freedom

This situation can also result in complications, whether the loss is temporary or permanent. Some of the freedom-restricted losses that can place people at risk include partial or total restrictions, as well as general life choice restrictions.

For example, the loss of freedom that follows forced hospitalization (whether acute or long term) and institutionalization (prisons, long-term care facilities) usually increases the risk factor for complications.

Likewise, the use of restraints (including personal restraining mechanisms such as walkers, wheelchairs, handcuffs, restraint devices, and seclusion experiences) is usually traumatic and contributes to complicated grief, even when this is a side effect of other losses.

Forced guardianships, or other powerful persons/situations, that limit one's own autonomy contribute to unsettling loss of freedom and can become a risk factor in developing complicated grief.

Dependency (inability to do care for self, inability to drive, restriction to smaller living space that is not considered one's own, reliance on persons for basic needs, socialization, and pleasure) can also be a factor placing a person at risk for complications.

Loss Resulting in Undesirable Changes

Often the undesirable nature of a change may cause complications. This is particularly so if the required change goes against one's self-image, beliefs, and values. These changes may increase anxiety. The person may feel devalued and fear sharing feelings.

Some changes are accomplished straightforwardly, yet others meet with great resistance. For these reasons, resistance to change must always be addressed contextually to determine the effect this resistance has on making healthy changes. In some cases, a person may feel that his or her values and beliefs may be placed in jeopardy by making a change that seems desirable to others. At other times, the change may have additional concrete and far-reaching implications.

For example, the death of a beloved grandmother who had a happy and fulfilling life can leave one deeply saddened. In this situation one might not expect such a loss to result in formidable changes and complicated grief. However, a loss such as this can lead to changes that affect everyday functioning. Sometimes the death of a grandmother means the loss of housing, the loss of financial and emotional support, and the loss of wisdom and guidance. Sometimes the loss of a grandmother is similar to the loss of a parent, resulting in overwhelming and unwelcomed changes. Who could argue about the undesirability of such a loss on a person who is developmentally not ready to stand independently.

Losses that are also internally traumatic can lead to a diminished sense of self.

- This type of loss can include loss of jobs or vocations that are considered an integral part of self—such as is often the case with clergy, police officers, teachers, and politicians.

- The loss of children due to reaching adulthood and leaving home, can occasionally become the source of complicated grieving, particularly when the children are the source of identity and focus for a marriage or understanding of oneself.
- The loss of health, aging, or retirement can be undesirable and present a threat to how one sees oneself. Retirement can be looked forward to but still, in practice, be undesirable due to the changes that come in role and context in society.

Any of these experiences can bring about the feeling of loss of self and/or loss of identity. Such loss is frequently complicated to some degree. Whenever a significant loss of identity occurs it may be a symptom of unhealthy dependency, highly enmeshed relationships, developmental functions that are not as advanced as would be desirable, or developmental tasks that must be undertaken.

Finally, on a different note, some changes are never experienced as desirable or acceptable. Failure to make changes can place a person at risk for complications and dysfunction. Such circumstances may result in long-term unresolved grief, impoverished quality of life, or in the need to put compensatory effort in less significant changes that one is willing to make. The challenge here is that resentment and bitterness can linger and become a barrier to natural growth and wellness.

Multiple Losses

Whenever a story begins with a string of losses, it is a good idea to delve deeper into each personal experience. However, while taking a careful loss history, one must remind the person that it is actually not uncommon to have multiple losses that can occur over a lifetime or over a brief period of time. However, when difficulty in health or in coping and multiple losses are experienced (no matter how close in chronology those losses are), the person needs to know that he or she is at risk for complications and for possible impairment in functioning. Of course this risk means that it is always wise to get professional input and to become as educated about grief as possible.

Betrayals

Complications often arise when loss is experienced as betrayal. The experience of betrayal can involve secrets, loss of financial security, abuse, or lead to divorce. The betrayal does not necessarily have to be proven. Rather it must be believed to have occurred to be experienced as loss and to place one at risk for grief. When the betrayal has not occurred, it is anticipatory grief. The betrayal does not need to be concrete. It can involve not living up to expectations or going against values that were once highly prized. As with other losses, betrayals are sorted out though the depression stage of grief, where they can be put in perspective and even discarded if unfounded.

Dramatic betrayals can complicate grief and transform people who successfully move through it. In the following example, the transformation was one of loss of innocence about personal safety and honorable conduct. Those who recovered understood that their view could no longer be considered the only view in the larger world community and that a return to the old could never happen again if they were to face this new reality.

In this example, the brutal killing of Daniel Pearl in Pakistan following the terrorist attacks on New York and Washington on September 11, 2001, was in some ways a betrayal of a code of ethics that we, the grieving people back home, thought governed action even during war. The death was videotaped and made available to the world, and the brutality of the killing significantly increased a general outrage and fear resulting from this type of death. This fear had a greater intensity than the death of other soldiers who were engaged in what was considered to be an honorable battle.

Stigmatic and Shaming Losses

Almost all stigmatic losses lead to an initial sense of shame that can complicate grief. However, losses do not have to be socially stigmatic (e.g., developing AIDS or having a mental illness) to be experienced as shameful. Being shamed is experienced as a result of external conditions, forces, or responses, and therefore becomes an additional assault or trauma in an already traumatic circumstance.

The risk for complication is greater for a person experiencing a stigmatic loss. A stigmatic loss is by definition a shaming experience from the larger community perspective. When a stigma is involved, even accepting resources is risky. Often an individual feels the need to hide anything about the lost object, person, or relationship. This kind of risk always involves the fear of exposure and/or ridicule that comes at already vulnerable times.

Personal Factors or Condition of the Survivor

Many personal factors that relate to the grieving person's condition, or the survivor, have the potential for increasing the risk for complications to develop during the course of grief. Some of these factors or conditions have been included in previous categories. This is because it is impossible to truly separate factors that are integrated within one's self and one's relational environment. In this case, the focus is not completely on the relationship or on the nature or essence of the loss itself. More attention is now directed to the internal state and functioning of the person who has suffered the loss. Some of the high-risk conditions that a survivor or grieving person might encounter as a result of loss are:

Current Health

When energy needed for the maintenance of one's own health is instead used for the processing of grief, it can cause a depletion of energy resources and increase the risk for development of complications.

Ability to Learn

Individuals with learning difficulties also have increased vulnerability in terms of processing grief. It may actually take too much energy for slower learners to try to understand what has happened. They may have difficulty knowing their own feelings. It may be very difficult to make changes or even know what changes need to be made. Those who have problems learning tend to experience great anxiety and may become overwhelmed, panicked, or depressed. Those who learn more quickly tend to move through grief more rapidly, barring other factors.

Readiness

Previous experiences with complicated or dysfunctional grieving may inhibit one's general readiness to respond to loss and the consequent experience of the pain and challenge of grief. One is never really ready for loss but successful recovery experiences help to build faith, hope, and confidence in the ability to grieve without becoming completely overwhelmed. Nothing increases readiness to face whatever life brings so much as having personal knowledge that one is able to do so.

Inhibiting Factors

Numerous inhibiting factors within a person may complicate grief. As mentioned previously, learning challenges and personal health issues inhibit some people so much that their functioning becomes impaired. Persons with personality factors that prevent them from taking risks will encounter more difficulty getting through ordinary events in functional ways.

Some people develop so many inhibiting factors that they create strong internal censors that may cause them to be inhibited. A personality plagued by inhibitions is also plagued by fears. This personality is often chained to rituals, regardless of their productivity and usefulness in meeting personal needs. Therefore, severely inhibited people do not handle new events well.

Instead, a new event is made to conform to the person's normative responses for all events. The problem is clear when one remembers that every loss is a new experience. A life plagued by unproductive restrictions restrains the authentic self. This makes it challenging for such a person to meet new experiences with a genuine desire to understand, survive, and grow.

Involvement in Familial and Communal Issues

It has not been determined that greater involvement with others is a factor for decreasing the risk for complicated grieving. However, experience dictates that perceived involvement and connection aids in recovery. Perceived lack of connection has the opposite effect of enhancing loss and disconnection.

Attitudes and Beliefs

Attitudes and beliefs are the sparks of the spirit that motivate human endeavors. When these sparks are not working we are at risk for breaking down. Although grief involves doubt and ambivalence about beliefs, those whose beliefs and attitudes have not been tested, have been found lacking, or are in need of revision or reconfirmation are at greater risk than those who have taken the opportunity to engage in this spiritual growth.

Inner Resources

In general, one's total being is engaged in the grief process when loss occurs. All parts need to work together in ways that nurture and complement one another. However, some latitude exists for the mind to take a break, for feelings to come and go, for the spirit to question and doubt, and even for an outbreak of a horrendous case of the flu. Still, all of an individual's inner resources are essential for normal grief to be successful. Plus, there actually is a requirement for an equal displacement of the grief workload over time. The complete breakdown of one resource is not tolerable and causes complications. An extended breakdown will result in impairment that may become quite risky.

Character

The virtues many of us learned in childhood and throughout our life are crucial to successful grieving. These virtues are the foundations of our identity, our relational code, and our spiritual life. Primary virtues may vary in their use by individuals; nevertheless the lack of certain character elements contribute to a greater risk for complicated grief. Some essential virtues are honesty, respect, altruism, responsibility, and courage. Usually each person possesses one to three critically important virtues. The inability to exhibit these virtues at important moments threatens one's moral and spiritual life and is poorly tolerated in the long run.

Resources Available

Along with personal factors, resource factors have a crucial impact on the course of grief. When positive resources are available, complications can be addressed earlier using appropriate skilled intervention. Although resources are usually available to everyone, some resources are not the best choices for some people.

Negative resources include the following:

Alcohol and drugs
Work that takes over rest of life
Advice that interferes with grieving
Risk-taking ventures
Aggressive or violent action

Positive resources that can be helpful:

Prayer
Meditation
Self-help reading about grief
Appropriate exercise
Supervised medication
Good diet
Supportive friends

When grief becomes complex two types of resources seem most helpful. Within these two types of resources one will find a range of availability depending on where one lives, personal preference, finances, or insurance. Helpful professionals and support groups are crucial resources for managing and working through complicated grief.

Helpful Professionals

The first layer of helpful people is usually family and friends. As complications develop, the second layer of resources is often professional persons in the community who are not necessarily therapists but rather are chosen for their people skills and for their perceived supportive role. Such professionals include family doctors, primary care providers, teachers, clergy, employee assistance program personnel, and supervisors. The third layer of professional resources involves those who are trained in working with complicated grief.

Bereavement Support Groups

The first layer of supportive groups tends to be social groups, church groups, and special interest groups such as weight-loss groups, and other clubs and organizations. Those whose grief is profound and sometimes complicated are often referred to support groups. These groups are now available to most people and are usually homogeneous, based on the loss anticipated or experienced. The third layer of resources, for those whose grief is complicated, is a therapeutic group.

PEOPLE WHO ARE PARTICULARLY AT RISK

Many people are at risk for experiencing complicated grief. However, some people can be identified as being at higher risk than others (see also Appendix C). As stated previously, this does not mean that people in these categories will develop complications consequent to experiencing loss. Rather, these people are vulnerable when loss occurs.

Individuals with Multiple Losses

The sheer number of losses that happen simultaneously or during a brief time (one to three years) can be problematic. More than one loss that has previously been complicated can put an individual at risk for having difficulties with the next grieving process. At least one or more of these losses needs to be significant but after that, the impact of a few additional lesser losses will feel more significant than at other times.

For example, Lydia tells the story of her mother's struggle to recover from the big move to Florida. She is telling the story because she struggles to explain to her husband why it was so problematic for her mother to choose a new doctor. From her husband's point of view this is not an important issue. However, Lydia remembers her mother's grief regarding feeling uprooted at the time of her father's retirement.

When her father turned sixty-five he made the decision to retire to Florida. He chose a house, had it built, and announced to his wife that they were moving. Her mother was in shock. She had intended to work for another ten years and she would now be far away from her friends, her children, and her grandchildren. However, she moved with her husband. Once she arrived in Florida all the small tasks that needed to be done were too much for her. Now, ten years later, Lydia says that she doesn't think her mother has yet recovered. To complicate matters, her father has a fear of flying and has no interest in driving back to see people.

Individuals with Extensive Loss History, Particularly at Vulnerable Periods

Certain periods in an individual's life are more vulnerable for significant loss. Children are vulnerable to early loss of parents, instability of environment, illness, and traumatic experiences. Young adults are particularly vulnerable to multiple losses that may begin in childhood and continue in early adult years. Challenging losses for young adults can include problems with higher education, jobs, relationships, and major illnesses. Older adults often feel vulnerable when they need to move from their home, when they experience declining health, when they don't feel they are contributing to the community or to their family or that their values are appreciated. Often these cumulative losses during a vulnerable time lead to despair and hopelessness.

Individuals Who Have Experienced Severe Trauma

Trauma always puts an individual at risk for complicated grief. Severe trauma can lead to post-traumatic stress disorder that is an indication of complicated and dysfunctional grief. In assessing the impact of trauma on an individual's grieving process, it is important to remember that trauma occurs as a unique experience, just as a loss is a loss if a person declares it to be so. It is also crucial to remember that trauma is defined as an experience in which the individual feels overwhelmed and that his or her life is threatened. This, combined with a sense of hopelessness and helplessness, completes the traumatic event. It is not necessary to be the direct recipient of a traumatic threat to be traumatized by the experience of witnessing such an event.

Individuals Whose Loved One Died a Violent, Horrendous, or Unfathomable Death

Violent, horrendous, or unfathomable deaths also put an individual at risk for complicated grieving. As one young woman stated, "I probably never should have heard all the details of my cousin's death or seen the police pictures at the trial. I can't get them out of my mind." Her cousin had been raped and murdered as a teenager. She was very close to her cousin's age and spent a lot of time with her cousin. To make matters worse, she had always looked to her cousin for support and help and felt that loss too. A further complication developed when she couldn't attend the funeral, and it was a long time before she was in any condition to visit her cousin's graveside. But the worst challenge came when she attended the trial and saw the photos of her dead cousin.

Individuals with Concurrent Mental Illness, Particularly Depression and Anxiety

People who have mental illness are capable of grieving in a normal manner. However, when a loss that coincides with episodes of acute depression or anxiety, the person is at additional risk for complicated grief. People who are actively psychotic at a time of profound loss may also have difficulty processing the loss until they are more mentally stable. Careful attention must be paid to the illness and the complications that it presents, as well as the other losses that may occur while the person is acutely ill.

Individuals with Impaired Personality Traits

Certain personality traits can present a risk for complicated grieving. People who have difficulty managing inner feelings in relational contexts often experience ambivalence over losses and are overwhelmed with feelings that they have difficulty expressing in appropriate ways. The loss of a person, object, or thing that an individual is very dependent on physically, socially, emotionally, and spiritually can become problematic due to the changes and chaos involved in such loss. Dependent personalities and those who have a borderline personality disorder have difficulty separating themselves from the lost object or person. Dependent individuals may not have the necessary skills for ordinary living and may become outraged when faced with learning to care for themselves. Those with borderline personality disorder are usually plagued by urges to be close to, and at the same time, distant, from others. People with narcissistic personality disorders run the risk of being personally wounded and inappropriately outraged when a significant loss occurs. Each personality disorder has its own implied vulnerability to loss and the consequent grief work.

Individuals Who Exhibit Extreme Defenses of Minimization and Globalization

Minimization involves the attempt to make a loss, or the effects of the loss less important. Globalization, on the other hand, is a response that magnifies the significance of a loss and makes global conclusions that may not stand the test of reality or reason. During normal grief processes both of these defenses may be used appropriately. These defenses are especially important during the denial and feelings stages when protection is needed to absorb the impact of the loss and to set a grief pace that is manageable. Ideally, individuals will alternate between the two responses before settling on an accurate assessment. Healthy truth often begins to emerge, built during the depressive stage of grief when real sorting occurs.

Underidentification or minimization of loss challenges the grief process because much energy must be expended to maintain the suppression of feelings. Yet, this minimization does not fool the person, so these feelings are still at work. The individual's energy acts much as acid does when it is churning and burning a hole through the stomach. Any control that one has through the mechanism of minimization is illusionary at best, for one is always at risk for these feelings coming to the surface.

Globalization of a loss is also an unstable response. When this defense is used, the grief response is greater than would otherwise be warranted. Even the grieving person experiences this drama as just a bit phony or overdone. But the compulsion to continue this type of dramatic response is pursued out of a desire to manage feelings of powerlessness, chaos, and a fear of being out of control. Authentic grief demands honesty and courage, not dishonesty and falseness. Globalization is a defense mechanism, used as a protection against guilt, shame, a genuine noncaring, or a fear of some other less acceptable grief response.

Isolated Individuals

Isolation is a risk factor for people experiencing loss. This does not mean that a person who lives alone is at greater risk. Rather, the greater risk is for the person who feels alone, feels cut off, or thinks he or she is without friends, family, and supportive people. Isolation can occur as a result of life events, certain illnesses, and personal choices. Because grief work needs to find expression for recovery to occur, isolation can limit the available forms of expression.

Individuals Contending with Real Guilt

It is a normal part of grief to wonder whether one is responsible for the loss that has occurred, and if responsible, how so. Feelings of guilt can be normal even when they prove unwarranted. One of the purposes of the internal sorting and review process is to ascertain what happened and the shifting nature of the relationship. In the midst of this process feelings of guilt are not necessarily problematic.

However those who experience guilt after a loss can become stuck in that feeling. Many people have actually said and done things that they feel were wrong, inappropriate, or that contributed to the loss. The nature and extent of the guilt will play a role in how these individuals manage their guilt in normal or complicated ways. In any case, it is crucial to remember that real guilt can be just as much a complication as false guilt. For these reasons it is imperative never to dismiss someone's guilt. A far better intervention is to help people sort through their guilt and reach their own conclusions. Both real and false guilt need resolution during the grief process, which is best conducted during the middle and latter part of depression and reorganization stages.

Individuals with Major Life-Skill Deficits

Major life-skill deficits can complicate life. In some cases the grief complication involves conceptually processing losses and changes. People with life-skill deficits need objective assessment of their daily functioning and specific plans in place to support skill growth or to support deficits that cannot be changed. The outcome of significant loss for individuals who have this challenge is positively enhanced by these quality supports.

Individuals Who Lose Children

Grief is always complicated by the loss of a child. However, recovery from grief may still be accomplished even if the resolution of loss looks different from other losses. It is important to understand and convey support to grieving parents for their depth of grief and pain. The risk is that parents may feel unsupported in their grief process and the choices they make to manage the loss of a child. Support groups have proven beneficial regarding the loss of a child. It is also helpful to find an appropriate time, usually long after the loss, to assure parents that their grief may take a long while to resolve. However, this does not mean that their grief will be constant or that their life will not have times of renewal. Here the notion of carrying one's grief needs to be used rather than focusing on the objective of recovery.

Sometimes a child does not die, but becomes developmentally or organically compromised. In these circumstances, parents face the loss of the child's unfulfilled potential. This circumstance is also a complication. The loss of an ideal child can be traumatic in its own way. However, families in this situation have a better chance for a more normal, albeit complicated, recovery, yet they must forever live with this situation.

Some of the complications in these circumstances can be addressed through homogeneous support groups that relate to the developmental level of the child.

For example, Joy's daughter was four years old when her mother took her once again to a doctor. Her daughter's speech was becoming more and more limited. She had reverted to crawling and seemed to develop unusual behaviors such as eating only food that was orange in color. After extensive testing, Joy was informed that her daughter was afflicted with autism, a permanent neurological disorder. Joy's grief process was complicated by the ever-present needs of her daughter and by her lack of knowledge about how to meet these needs. To her credit, she started a support group for people with similar needs. This group was helpful, however, the grief process of this family has yet to resolve itself.

ASSESSING COMPLICATED GRIEF TRAJECTORIES

Grief trajectories are paths that people take in their movement from loss to recovery (see Figure 1.1 in Chapter 1). A normal path generally moves somewhat sequentially through the six stages of grief. Yet, even within a normal path, a number of variations occur. This is also true for complicated grief. Therefore, complicated grief has its own template, or trajectory, that is used in addition to the normal stage template.

By using both normal and complicated grief templates, one is able to devise more accurate and more helpful treatment plans for those whose grief is complicated. Since people who are experiencing complicated grief respond well to being helped by professionals, it is crucial to use an assessment tool that will aid in the development of these concrete treatment plans with their corresponding appropriate interventions.

The Initial Process

The first step in the development of any grief trajectory begins with active listening to the story of loss. Asking the person to share how he or she is managing grief can follow this step. At some point it is also helpful to discuss the normal stages of grief to enlarge the person's understanding of where he or she is in this process.

If the grief is so acute that talking about the stages of grief is too overwhelming, then one can usually just cite the first three—shock, denial, and feelings. Those who are in the midst of strong feelings can sometimes only make it this far. The technique of going slowly when discussing stages of grief is always a good idea. Plus, it may be just as helpful to introduce the idea of stages after one's story has been told with, "I can understand how you were in shock and maybe still be just a bit overwhelmed." Presenting the gentle suggestion that grief is a process will help later on to lay a foundation for hopefulness that is essential to recovery. However, omit the introduction of stage and process theory whenever it is crucial to attend to the grief story and the feelings being presented.

Do what you can to keep individuals talking about the loss and their responses. Pay attention to general factors that may be present in the grief experience. Note whether the person falls into any high-risk categories. A mental comparison may also begin to develop between stage-specific issues that may have been completed and those that are still in process or have yet to begin.

The Search for Obstacles or Complications

With this type of information it is possible to continue with a more sequential assessment of grief processes. Although each grieving experience is unique, certain grief responses follow more complicated paths. Complicated grief trajectories are made up of responses defined by obstacles arising within the normal grief process. These obstacles usually stop, or drastically change, the course of grief. Whenever grief is considered complicated, one must look for the complications or obstacles that have developed.

Complications or obstacles are always manifested in one or more areas within the process and distort normal grief trajectories. By gathering information in four areas, the complication and distortion can be identified. A completed trajectory will contain the following:

1. Locus of complication
2. Stage-specific point of complication
3. Length of complication
4. Degree of complication

Trajectory Area 1:
Locus and Pervasiveness of Complication

The locus of distortion (obstacle, or complication) is addressed by assessing grief effects in one or more areas of human functioning. The helper's task is to find obstacles to the grief process within the grief story. To accomplish this task, one often needs to ask questions to gather more information from each area. Sometimes this approach can be supplemented by assessments used for depression or anxiety. Examples of locations of complications are as follows:

- *Physical obstacles:* Weight loss or heart pains
- *Psychological obstacles:* Minimization of loss or psychological wounding
- *Emotional obstacles:* Uncontrollable anger or fear

- *Social obstacles:* Separation from family or continued conflict with others
- *Spiritual obstacles:* Feelings of hopelessness or anger with God or power figures

Trajectory Area 2: Stage-Specific Point of Complication

Consideration of the normal stages of grief, and the tasks and issues that arise during those stages, helps in the assessment of stage-specific complications. By using information provided by the grieving person, and information gathered from resources such as presented in this book, one is able to identify problems within each stage. For example, a review of the grief process may show any of the following obstacles to normal grieving:

- *A loss factor:* Failure to attach to primary person who has died
- *A shock stage complication:* Recurrent nightmares of horrific type of death
- *A denial response:* Minimization of a significant relationship
- *Complicated feelings:* Continued rage or glorified love
- *Depression complications:* Continued apathy and lack of pleasure
- *Reorganization obstacles:* Refusal to make necessary adjustments
- *Recovery complications:* Vow to never care again

Trajectory Area 3: Length or Duration of Complication

Within each category of complicated grief, the trajectory as a whole could become distorted either temporarily, for a short duration, for a long time, or even permanently. But the use of time as a measure of normal versus complex grief is a complicated issue. In the past, it was often a temptation to set a specific time for the completion of a grief response. After that time expired, it was determined that grief was taking too long or lasting longer than usual. For deaths or divorces, the template for grief was one year. For loss of job or hospitalization, the time template might be generously extended to six months. To avoid this approach, which is often erroneous, it is best to note the date or time of loss and the length of time one has experienced the complication(s) described in trajectory areas 1 and 2. Thus, a grief trajectory may be said to be temporarily complicated, have a short-term complication, or evidence long-term complications.

- *Temporary Complications:* Three months of sleeplessness after the death of a spouse
- *Short-term complications:* One year of avoidance of going home after the loss of one's mother
- *Long-term complications:* Anger/rage and preoccupation with a former boss four years after being fired.

Trajectory Area 4: Degree or Severity of Complication

The degree of complication is assessed after gathering information in trajectory areas 1, 2, and 3. It is most helpful to make a decision of severity on a scale of 1 to 5. Some complications are close to the normal range and may be considered mild. These complications would be rated at 1 or 2. Other complications may cause more of a discomfort, or disruption in life pleasure, relationships, and activity, with moderate consequences. These would be rated at level 3. When severe complications significantly interfere with functioning, the degree rises to 4 or 5. These high-level ratings represent dysfunctional grieving or a high risk for dysfunctional grieving. In almost all cases, people with moderate complications would benefit from brief therapy. Those with severe complications usually need increased health care services.

- *Normal:* Yelling at son to clean up his room one morning
- *Mild (1-2):* Intermittent tears the few weeks following a cancer diagnosis
- *Moderate (3):* Twenty percent reduction in product output the six months after a miscarriage
- *Severe (4-5):* Refusal to look for work one year after loss of job

A Grief Trajectory Worksheet

For the helper's convenience, a Grief Trajectory Worksheet is located in Appendix D. This form can be used for assessing both complicated and dysfunctional grief. By using this tool one can readily assess grief process problems and determine what additional information is needed. One can also begin to pinpoint the basic elements to focus on for targeted interventions and for the development of a treatment plan. This form can be used for both brief care and counseling situations.

In addition to the use of a typical flow chart, there is also a place for providing the same material in a process format, i.e., the grief trajectory template focusing on the stage/journey of grief (located at the bottom of the form). Of course it is important to bear in mind that grief is not static or rigidly sequential, but rather is living and dynamic. So, a grief trajectory worksheet captures one moment in time for the purposes of analysis and reflection. The practice of reviewing the sheet helps to show progress and to quickly note unfinished work.

The grieving person, as well as the professional, could use such a worksheet. Ideally, the sheet could be completed collaboratively. However, do not ask a person who is overwhelmed with complications and who has not moved through the affect stage of grief to do the worksheet. Rather, gather information in the context of his or her story. In cases of significant complications, the grieving person will have difficulty completing such a sheet and will continue to need the catharsis that talking about grief provides. At minimum, those experiencing grief can usually name some of the problems they are experiencing and answer the question of approximately how long this problem has persisted.

Assessment of Complications Process Summary

In summary, the worksheet pulls together the information discussed in this chapter. The loss or losses are identified first. The grief story is told. A tentative history of losses is noted. In this case the history-taking process is open ended with ample opportunity to talk about losses that the person considers important. After this, complications are noted in terms of dimensions affected, stages affected, duration, and severity of complications.

During this assessment one can substitute any of these words for complication: obstacle, problem, or impairment. For complicated grief the words obstacle or problem are appropriate. As we shall see in the next chapter, for dysfunctional grief the word impairment is best used.

At the bottom of the worksheet the grief trajectory template of completed stages is circled. For stages to be successfully completed complications/impairments need to have returned to a low-moderate level or it is recorded that no complications are now noted in the severity column. While functioning can be mildly impaired, it should not be assessed as being far into the moderate zone or be considered of severe intensity. In addition, the functioning must not continue to significantly interfere with necessary daily activities.

The Grief Response Service Wheel

The goal of treatment for complicated and dysfunctional grief is to help the bereaved person (family) return to functional (albeit painful) grieving. In order to fulfill this goal, it is important to understand what grieving looks like along the continuum of normal, complicated, and dysfunctional responses. In Appendix E this continuum is presented in a circle form called a grief response service wheel.

By using this visual imagery one is able to see the relationship between the differing grief responses and to see the corresponding treatment goal and type of treatment intervention. Keep this service wheel in mind when making assessments and referrals for it provides the broader context in which providers and professionals work.

MORE EXPERIENCES OF COMPLICATED GRIEVING

The following vignettes are useful because they continue to give voice to the experiences of people whose grief processes are complicated. As such, they build empathy and understanding and remind us why we do this work. However, they can also be used to practice sharpening assessment skills and to try out the Grief Trajectory Worksheet (Appendix D).

It Can't Be Happening to Me

Guy was referred for grief counseling. He was a grieving teenager who had lost his father several years ago. He did not want to talk. He said, "I can't believe it even happened. It shouldn't have happened. I have no idea who did it. Why did this have to happen to me?" His father had been murdered, and Guy found his body lying in the street. Immediately he went home for help.

"I'm fine; I can take care of myself," he declares. Yet, his mother says that even though Guy has received counseling his anger is still great. He is becoming unmanageable. She knows he has become involved with drugs and alcohol. He sleeps all day and is failing at school. When she tries to talk to him, he yells at her and storms out of the house.

A Heart Hanging in Sorrow

Judith arrives in dark clothes. Everything about her is dark and brooding. She does not complete the intake form beyond writing her name, address, and phone number. When asked about her work she says, "It doesn't matter." She doesn't know why she has come for therapy, except that the pastor told her she should. She doesn't feel she has any strengths and says she supposes she has been depressed most of her adult life.

Yet Judith works at a job she has held for twenty-five years. She owns her own house and drives a car. She goes to church but does not participate outside of worship. She does not celebrate holidays and prefers to not spend much time with her aging mother. She says she has no hobbies. When asked about what might have brought on this depression she stares at her hands that are very still. "When I was twenty-two, I lost my husband in a hunting accident. He was my soul mate." She stops and says, "Can we stop now?"

Psychological Homelessness

In the movie, *Sarah, Plain and Tall: Winter's End* (1999) Jacob's father returns to the farm in Kansas. Jacob, who was a child when his father suddenly left him and his mother, is shocked. He thought his father was dead all these years. He is angry at being abandoned and about the consequent difficult years growing up with his mother and without a dad.

The father, John, came home knowing that he might die soon. At first he does not share his illness with his son. John says he had a yearning to see "how things turned out."

As the drama unfolds, John is encouraged to speak of his life after leaving his family and the farm some decades earlier. In the midst of his story of wandering from place to place for a minimum of thirty years, he declares, "I've never called any other place home." Later he says, "I've never found any other people to love." He had left the land because of the struggles and losses he felt in relationship to his wife who did not share his love of the land or the lifestyle that was important to him. He felt she blamed him for both, and that she and his son would be better off without him.

Shackles and Other Bindings

There are four people in an admissions recovery group. For the newcomers, we focus on identification of losses. For some this is an easy task. Marion is readily able to identify her losses. In fact, she has had so many losses that she becomes overwhelmed and lost in their identification and in the images that follow each one's description. Her most troublesome loss is that she is a survivor of incest.

Marion's overidentification with loss has been managed in the group by encouraging her to practice reflective observation by noticing and reporting her thoughts and the feelings that arise as a result of these thoughts. When she tends to become overwhelmed by her feelings and sink into depression, or spring into anger, she is encouraged to choose a transition exercise that would help her. Often she chooses to take a deep breath and exhale or to completely change the subject. At times she is directed to focus on her losses one by one, beginning with the least troublesome ones.

However, under stress Marion moves rather quickly to an experience of overwhelming loss. Today she states, "I'm not afraid of dying; I am afraid of living." She is being discharged in one week and will go back to her apartment and her life. She says her overwhelming feeling is of being "scared." She feels bound or controlled by her past. We talk about her ambivalent thoughts. Today these thoughts are examples of the denial she is trying to use as a protective shield. This denial fluctuates from one extreme to another—"It will be all right," or "It will be all bad and disastrous."

A Loss of Self

Cherie requests a visit from the chaplain, whom she has never met. She is short and overweight. Her age is not obvious. She could be in her late twenties or early thirties. She begins by taking the chaplain to her room and showing her pictures she is cutting out for collages. All the pictures are of beautiful, elegantly dressed women doing exciting things that suggest an abundant lifestyle. We go to another room for more privacy. She brings out a scrapbook and a package of pictures. She begins to go through her pictures, identifying the individuals for the chaplain. She does the same with the scrapbook. Mostly she chronicles her junior and senior high school years. She was a thin, pretty, active, and involved teen. Her name and her picture are clearly displayed in print several times.

At the end of this sharing Cherie declares, "They don't believe me. They don't think I am the person in these pictures. They don't think I was pretty or that I had lots of friends. I keep trying to tell them that I am this person. "

Since her teen years Cherie has had more than one experience of "breaking down." She looks far older than her current years, although she is clearly not yet middle aged. She is currently hospitalized in a psychiatric facility.

Where to Begin to Grieve

Lara has a sister who is terminally ill with cancer. Over the course of several conversations she talks about this sister who lives on the other coast. Lara is concerned. She feels that her sister is vulnerable because she is not doing what Lara feels would be helpful to manage her illness. "She is listening to strangers," Lara says, "people who are currently in her life and who may be taking advantage of her." She is using new age, homeopathic efforts rather than relying on her medical doctors.

Lara and her sister talk to each other several times a week. Lara feels that her sister and her sister's illness are consuming her whole life. Lara is distraught and wants to have some kind of book that can help her deal with her grief.

We talk again. This time I suggest that Lara not treat her sister as "her ill sister" but rather as a whole person. That may be the best gift she can give to her sister, her family, and herself. Several months later, Lara informs me that my suggestion was helpful. Then she tells me that her sister died. She bursts into tears. She cannot sleep. She cannot focus. She has difficulty being civil to colleagues. She is yelling at her family. "I just don't know where to begin to grieve," she declares.

Beginning Life with Loss

Sam, who is in a wheelchair, has a speech impediment but is able to speak somewhat clearly. His loss is stated in terms of loss of "liberty" from being at the hospital and of losing control of his life. He says he isn't afraid of living but he is angry about all the losses that he has experienced due to cerebral palsy. He admits that he also "has a temper" that can get out of control. Finally, he says that "his loss began at birth." He seems almost surprised to hear himself say this but he remains quiet after the statement and lets others talk. When the group is finished he leaves rather quietly, which is a change from his usually upbeat departure.

SUMMARY

Loss is an everyday part of life and grief is a universal response to loss. Even so, grief can become overwhelming and complicated. These experiences of complication bring people to health providers, clergy, and therapists, as well as to other professionals in the helping field. In all cases, individuals having difficulty recovering from loss have a personal and unique story to tell about what has happened to them, how they are facing the loss or losses, and where they are experiencing difficulty.

Helping another person manage grief is not an easy process. It requires compassion, skill, and a willingness to enter the pain-filled world of grief and be companion to the individual on his or her path to recovery. Sometimes, it is difficult for people to identify where they feel overwhelmed or stuck. Sometimes, people don't even know that they are having problems with their grief. In all cases, it is helpful for the professional to know stage-specific complications that can arise, general factors that affect grieving and may cause complications, as well as categories of people who are particularly at risk for developing complications.

With this knowledge and careful listening to the grieving person, it is possible to understand the path that grief is taking for that person.

It is possible to develop a clinical picture of the grief experience and to identify and even predict possible complications in the future. These skills benefit the griever. When services are developed collaboratively with knowledgeable, skilled, and compassionate professionals, people are more apt to experience some resolution to complications, change dysfunctional behaviors, and return to a more normal course of grieving.

Chapter 3

Dysfunctional Grieving

Be merciful to me, O God,
be merciful to me,
for in thee my soul takes refuge;
in the shadow of thy wings
I will take refuge,
till the storms of destruction pass by.

Psalm 57:1

A young woman spoke with her doctor. She was having problems with relationships. She was using drugs. They weren't the hard-core drugs, but nevertheless she needed them. She had been brought to the hospital against her wishes. During the conversation with her new doctor she tearfully explained that she was having problems because she missed her mother, who had died. The doctor was empathetic and understood the grief that follows the death of one's mother. He listened and asked questions about her health and her lifestyle. However, as the conversation continued he began to wonder about the mother's death. So he asked, "When did your mother die?" "Five years ago," she said sadly. "That's why I'm here today and why all of this is happening to me."

As a result of this intake interview, the doctor referred the young woman for grief counseling, saying, "There's a lot of grieving going on inside. At first I thought it was a recent loss. I was surprised to find out that the loss happened five years ago. I think she might benefit from the loss and recovery group and maybe from some individual attention."

This kind of referral is common. Dysfunctional responses to grief are often discovered while addressing problems that seem to have no overt link to grief. However, further inquiry into the presenting problem and condition frequently suggests that roots of many problems are embedded in loss and aggravated by challenging grief processes. In many instances, it is not unusual for the grieving person or close family and friends, to trace the onset of current problems back to a specific significant loss or a combination of losses.

Whether or not a helper is taking a detailed loss history, initial tasks include listening to the presenting problem, asking questions, drawing out further information, and early formulation of a professional hypothesis as to what is going on and possible treatment/response options. In the case of grief problems, the initial inquiry focuses on losses and their effect. However, even when grief does not overtly bring the person to treatment, in the course of presenting their problems, people mention losses, or imply losses, when they talk about their life circumstances. In any case, when a specific loss is identified, or inferred, a hypothesis must be tentatively formulated about the relationship between the loss and the presenting problem. The most tenable hypothesis is that the problem may be an indication that grief has become complicated and that there may be some degree of impairment. The next tenable hypothesis is that grief may have aggravated a preexisting problem.

> An Assessment Rule of Thumb: When problems of any kind are evident, a loss and grief assessment should be conducted.

Whenever significant losses or changes occur, a more extensive loss history is important. To conduct these assessments, the helper needs to have developed ways of discerning at what point grief has stopped being normal, thus becoming complicated or dysfunctional.

THE INITIAL INQUIRY

To make this differential diagnosis, the initial inquiry needs to uncover the nature of each loss and the impact that it has on one's ability to cope. Where a number of significant losses occur, the impact is often cumulative. If so, further inquiries must focus on the cumulative impact of loss over time. Additional questions are asked to discern at what point coping mechanisms and grief responses might have gotten off track. After this, one must gather information about professional and less formal interventions that have been tried and determine the result of these interventions. This information will help determine other interventions that might be appropriate and effective. The earlier these investigative questions are asked, the greater the potential for positive intervention and beneficial outcomes.

The additional step of gathering information about previous interventions is very important to the success of future efforts. In Wilma's case this question helped her feel more hopeful about engaging in group therapy. Wilma was referred for loss and recovery therapy due to multiple losses. This was her first hospitalization. The day she finally appeared for group work she ended up in a small group with only one other person. That person had been a part of this group for six months and was quite willing to talk about her frustrations with a parent who was drinking again. Wilma said she had been without a drink for two weeks and she wanted one badly. Although she empathized with the other person she had no intentions of stopping. She found that the problems that seemed so great when she was sober were not so great when she was drunk. Given the choice, she'd rather stay drunk. The therapist was amazed that Wilma had shown up for this group session, as she had not attended any during the last two weeks. Upon further inquiry the therapist learned that Wilma had over thirty years of experience in working with professionals. It all began when she was identified as a child who needed help and would spend extra time talking with her teacher. Then there were successions of individual and group therapies. This help had proved useless and at her age she had no desire to change. When the group ended she confirmed that the next session would be in two days.

Early Formulation of Concepts and Terminology

Let us return to the formulation of concepts and terminology that aid in the assessment and treatment of grief processes. For as much as we would like an orderly process with a format similar to following a recipe in a cookbook, an essential back-and-forth movement occurs between theory, or concepts and practice, or application. To ask the questions and gather the information needed to decide what help a grieving person needs, one must decide which terms are used to describe which processes. Hence, specific definitions and terms in the early chapters of this book describe normal and complicated grieving. Now, terms and definitions must be selected to further clarify dysfunctional grief and its place in the continuum of grief responses. But selection of terminology for dysfunctional grieving is even more challenging than for normal grief.

LABELING GRIEF RESPONSES

In general, American society is somewhat confused about how to label grief responses. This is true at individual, familial, communal, and national levels even though rituals that promote healthy grieving can still be found. This confusion exists because grief is painful and we want to get through the process as quickly as possible. Even in the midst of a great variety of resources, we often choose to cross our fingers, maybe say a prayer, and do what we have to do. As a result, we remain in partial or complete denial about grief, in order to be about the business of recovery. The effects of our persistent denial can be both positive and negative. On the positive side, we are progressive, growth oriented, inventive, and strong. On the negative side, denial of grief has profound stress-inducing effects that catch us by surprise when we least expect them.

On September 11, 2001, terrorists used commercial jetliners to destroy the World Trade Centers in New York City and to fly into the Pentagon in Washington, DC. A fourth plane crashed in Pennsylvania before it could reach its intended destination, which was speculated to be either the White House or the Capitol. Thousands of innocent persons died that day. Thousands of friends and families were in shock, and millions of Americans and people from all over the world experienced grief. Yet, within just a few days President George W. Bush urged the citizens of the nation to get back to work. Citizens were told that it was a patriotic thing to do. By going about the business of working and buying things the country would be helped. More caution was encouraged. But the general theme was of getting on with our lives. We were to contribute to our country by not letting this loss get us down. We must show our strength. The call to almost instantaneous recovery was made before the extent of the devastation was fully known.

Yet, the terror and grief of that tragedy lives on in our country and in other parts of the world. In a small church, five months later, the pastor and congregation prayed for a member who was flying out of town for a planned vacation. They prayed for her safety. They sent her on the "wings of prayer." With shaky humor, some said they had never remembered praying so intently over a domestic airplane ride.

Ambivalence Abounds

A review of literature on complicated grief reveals that there is ambivalence about what to call any grief response that does not follow the commonly accepted "normal" course. For example, this recent quote from Nadine Melhem and colleagues in the journal article titled, " Co-morbidity of Axis I Disorders in Patients with Traumatic Grief," demonstrates this point. These authors state that pathologic grief has "often been referred to as 'complicated,' 'pathologic,' 'atypical,' 'neurotic,' or 'unresolved' grief." The authors then add their own term, "traumatic grief," to the list (Melhem et al., 2001, p. 884).

Others use these categories and more. The list has actually become rather exhaustive and a bit cumbersome. All names refer to a process of nonnormal grieving. Many times these labels are used interchangeably:

pathological	inhibited
atypical	distorted
traumatic	delayed
neurotic	absent
morbid	unresolved
dysfunctional	complicated

Although the uniqueness of each label can be defended as representative of processes occurring in some grief responses, a generally acceptable consensus regarding terminology has yet to be reached. This is a problem for clinicians and other helpers. For those engaged in treatment of complicated and dysfunctional grieving, a simple, yet descriptive and functional labeling system is needed.

A case for a consensus in terminology and the universality of assessment for complicated and dysfunctional grief can be illustrated anecdotally by reflection on clinical referrals. Some referrals are made for complicated grief when the grief is rather normal and uncomplicated. This means grief is sometimes considered dysfunctional even when an individual is actually functioning very well in a challenging situation.

Dysfunctional grief, on the other hand, is often considered pathological even when the dysfunction does not constitute an actual disease. So people referred for pathological grieving are not necessarily pathological in their grief, even though their grief may be complicated. At other times, the term pathological is used when referring to criminal behaviors that are part of an overall dysfunctional grief response, but are not necessarily disease based. Criminal behavior is certainly impaired behavior, but not necessarily evidence of disease in the strictest sense. Increased clarity regarding grief and grief responses would help provide greater accuracy in assessment, diagnosis, and treatment.

Toward Simplification of Grief Terminology

In the context of this work, three major categories of grief responses are identified. In Chapter 1, the normal grief response was reviewed. In Chapter 2, the complications of grief were discussed with the inclusion of a second category for complicated grieving. In this chapter dysfunctional behaviors are described, and the third category of dysfunctional grieving is added. Normal grief, complicated grief, and dysfunctional grief are used when they refer to an overall pattern of response. Otherwise, processes and components within these patterns are being discussed.

The processes and components within the overall grief pattern are important, for each grief response has within it the potential for complications (factors and conditions that are part of the whole grief response). In addition, each response has within it the potential for dysfunctional thinking, feelings, and behaviors that may lead to increasing degrees of disorder and impairment. Thus, normal grieving patterns, complications, and areas of dysfunction are all taken into consideration in determining whether individual grief responses are normal, complicated, or dysfunctional. An accurate determination of the general grief response based on identifiable complications and dysfunctions helps promote preventative processes and provision of interventions that increase the likelihood for better recovery outcomes. Because this is somewhat complex to conceptualize, Table 3.1 is included here to provide a crisp format for understanding these three grief responses and their components.

TABLE 3.1. Grief Responses

	Normal Grief	Complicated Grief	Dysfunctional Grief
Grief Response			
Response: refers to overall pattern or process of movement of grief from loss through recovery	Refers to typical grief response patterns for most persons	Refers to complexity of grief response Making the response not as typical as otherwise expected	Grief responses that are evidenced by impairment, disease, inappropriate actions, drastic/life threatening, and perhaps criminal consequences
Complications			
Complications refer to grief complexity, i.e., factors and conditions that are part of the whole grief response	Minimal problems in recovering from loss Mild complications may be present Minimal dysfunction may happen but does not persist	Severity of complications: Mild Moderate Severe May impede grief response Complicated grief may lead to disorder and/or impairment	Severity of complications: Mild Moderate Severe Complications may lead to dysfunctions and dysfunctions may increase complications
Dysfunction			
Dysfunction refers to the grief response impairment Degree of impairment, i.e., the effects and actions as a result of impairment of grief process	Minimal Mild Dysfunction usually transient Adaptations made as a result of adequate coping skills and availability and use of resources	Mild Moderate Severe Interventions are often helpful to address or prevent dysfunction from occurring. Complications that have moderate or severe consequences usually need professional help	Mild Moderate Severe Typical areas of impairment a. Disease (Pathology) b. Destructive processes and behaviors

When Complications Become Barriers

Grief is a challenge even when the loss does not involve factors and conditions that cause impaired responses. However, some losses do become overwhelming. When this occurs, challenges turn into complications that become obstacles, and then barriers. Once barriers to the grief process occur, possibility increases for intense dysfunction in the form of health problems, disease, and other destructive processes and behaviors. A barrier is built when a challenge or problem has become a complication or obstacle that cannot be worked through. The severity and rigidity of a barrier makes it a major criterion in a dysfunctional grief response.

Definition of Dysfunctional Grieving

At the simplest level, dysfunctional grieving is made up of a combination of thoughts, feelings, and actions that are not working productively toward recovery. So, dysfunctional grieving is a significantly disordered or impaired grief response.

It is this nonproductive response that often indicates significant barriers to the recovery process, and these barriers keep the person stuck in grief. Although it is true that during mild and moderately complicated grief one may need to make adaptations in order to function while still grieving, this is no longer the case when grief takes a dysfunctional turn. For when the grief process is predominantly dysfunctional, adaptations are not made and functioning starts to break down. In some cases, former functioning (functioning prior to the loss) may not return. Certainly, the more dysfunctional the grief, the more sophisticated professionals need to be with their interventions.

LOCUS OF IMPAIRMENT

Dysfunction can be determined by assessing areas where impairment may be manifested. These areas are located internally, externally, and in transcendent and transpersonal realms. Each location relates to different functions. Holistic care requires assessment in physical (including mental), psychological, social, and spiritual areas. Although described separately, these are structural ways of describing interconnected and complex areas. Once structurally separated, impairment can be more accurately identified.

The locus of impairment can also be described contextually. In this approach, areas of human functioning are further clustered as located primarily internally, externally, or in transcendent/transpersonal groupings. This clustering approach focuses on the primary source of dysfunction rather than on affected areas.

Internal Impairments

- Physical/biological area
- Psychological area
- Personal spiritual area

Careful attention to an individual's thinking process, range, and quality of feelings is part of identifying the locus of function or dysfunction. Thought processes can be impaired, just as moods can be appropriate or disordered. Focus must be on the continuum of thoughts and feelings, including their presence or notable absence. It is crucial to gather data about thoughts, feelings, actions, and beliefs that were typical prior to a loss, during a loss, and following a loss.

Internal impairment often crosses over the individual areas of internal impairment. Chip experienced this problem after his mother died. He was in charge of setting up funeral services, making burial arrangements, executing her will, arranging the sale of her house, and keeping his three brothers and sister from fighting with one another. Everyone agreed that he did a wonderful job. You could see tears in his eyes now and then, and he sometimes seemed to have his mind elsewhere, but he came through with flying colors.

A year after his mother's death, Chip started to have chest pains and was rushed to the hospital. The stress test showed no heart difficulties, so he let it go at that. Two months after the stress test his boss noted that Chip didn't seem to be himself lately. When asked to elaborate, his boss said he didn't know how to pinpoint the change, but observed that Chip didn't seem to have the same old initiative, or drive, that he once had. He didn't seem to respond as quickly. Shortly after that, Chip's wife wondered if he was OK and suggested he see a doctor. It didn't really matter one way or another to Chip, but he said he would make an appointment with his primary care doctor. When the time came to go he forgot and as an explanation said he couldn't remember making such an appointment. The last straw, from his wife's point of view, came when he stopped going to church, saying he'd rather stay home and sleep.

That was when Chip's wife insisted he go see his doctor and arranged to go with him. After carefully listening to Chip, and to his wife, the doctor referred Chip to a therapist. It took only one session for the therapist to hypothesize that these problems might have internal sources, even though their effects were growing more widespread. Chip was referred to a psychiatrist who recommended an antidepressant. Meanwhile, he was referred to a pastoral psychotherapist who was trained in grief therapy, and could also relate to Chip's spiritual distress that seemed to appear as a result of the loss of his mother.

External Impairments

Social/relational areas:
• Family and significant others
• Friends and acquaintances
• Community and culture

When the locus of impairment is in the external context of intimate as well as extended relationships, it can be helpful to speak, with the person's permission, with others who will be able to describe functioning and impairment from their perspective. Of course, this information could also be used to describe manifestations of internal processes, as well as observations of behavior, communication, and changes in relational processes and espoused beliefs.

In Charles' case, his brother's suicide left him holding the bag. Not only was he grieving the loss of his brother, but also his brother's death complicated everything. Louis was an outgoing and affectionate guy most of the time. When he was in a good mood, Louis was on top of the world. When he was having a hard time, he seemed to be in the pits. This is the way it had been as long as Charles could remember. Throughout his adult life Louis was in and out of hospitals for bipolar disorder. Charles had finally come to grips with the mental illness, and the fact that Louis' health always seemed to be on a roller coaster.

Charles was angry about the wake of problems Louis left behind. The bills were sky high and Louis' family had no support income after Louis died. Louis had five children from two different mothers, and now everyone was coming to Charles for help. To make matters worse, it wasn't easy to tell the church that Louis had committed suicide, and the close-knit community in which they had both lived all their lives didn't seem to understand. It became so painful seeing old friends on the street that Charles began to avoid them. In fact, he even put his house on the market and thought it would be better if he left town.

This is when Charles' pastor stepped in and confronted him. Once the pastor saw the For Sale sign, he knew something had to be done. He had heard others talking about Charles' avoidance behavior but he chalked it up to grief, deciding that it was normal to be a little out of sorts. However, selling his house so suddenly and moving away was another thing. Later on, Charles said what really helped him was the pastor calling him on the phone and insisting on coming over to see him. This was the first time in many months that Charles was able to talk about the effects that Louis' suicide had on him. The pastor followed up with two other appointments, after which Charles took his house off the market and began talking to a few close friends.

Transcendent/Transpersonal Impairments

- Spiritual area

Assessing and focusing on transcendent/transpersonal impairments is often challenging. This is particularly so when a person does not express distress in the spiritual area. Without explicit direction from the person in distress, professionals may shy away from being what they consider intrusive in private matters. Even when impairment may be obviously coming from spiritual distress, or have affected spiritual practices, there is a tendency to address other areas more aggressively. Sometimes no formal intervention is made unless the spiritual stress is identified as part of a larger disease pattern, such as mental illness. When this is the case, the spiritual issue becomes subsidiary to what is considered the primary issue.

Joan was a good Baptist. She was not overly religious, but enjoyed believing that she was a good person in good standing with her church. She believed that her life had been better since she had been baptized and accepted Christ as her personal savior.

Joan was not pushy about her religion. She never argued with people inside her church or otherwise. She respected all beliefs, even if she did not personally agree with them. In a way, she was a bit old-fashioned, and accepted what she heard in church with a grain of salt. She couldn't see a need to convert or evangelize others.

This approach changed the moment she heard that her husband had cheated on her with another woman. At first, she could not believe it. She was a good Christian woman and he was a deacon in the church. Right away she went for therapy to manage her depression. She knew she was depressed when she couldn't get out of bed, didn't want to do anything, and wasn't able to work effectively. During therapy she discovered that it was difficult to forgive Richard, so she worked on this issue. Then she realized that she was stuck and really couldn't forgive herself for not realizing what was happening long ago. She could not dispel the recurring feeling that she didn't deserve to have Richard's love. In fact, she couldn't see how anyone could love her. One day, four years after the divorce, it dawned on Joan that she no longer believed there was a God. A friend, who was also a church member, suggested Joan go to a pastoral therapist but Joan saw no need. She died at the age of seventy-nine having never changed her mind.

SEVERITY OF IMPAIRMENT

In addition to locus of impairment, dysfunctional grief is also categorized by severity of impairment. As with complicated grief, a severity scale is useful. Using this scale, dysfunctional grief can be assessed as consisting of mildly, moderately, or severely impaired functioning.

Severity Scale

- *Mildly Dysfunctional*
  - Intermittent impairment
  - Transitory
  - Able to continue basic functions
  - Small coping adaptations
- *Moderately Dysfunctional*
  - Some diminishment of basic functions for longer period of time

- • Crucial life functions continued
- • Challenged coping in specified areas
- • *Severely Dysfunctional*
  - • Problems with performing basic functions, including life skills
  - • Crucial life functions threatened
  - • Adaptation abilities diminishing

Even the grief from a single trauma can result in differing degrees of dysfunctional responses. Mildly dysfunctional responses may be categorized as dysfunctional grieving, or they may be considered part of complicated grieving. This could be so if the impairment is limited and the effects are not pervasive.

For example, a person who had a significant car accident on a four-lane highway may avoid driving on such highways for years after the accident. If there is no reason that the person has to drive on a four-lane highway, then the dysfunctional behavior may be an inconvenience, or complication, but not a large problem.

As a result of the same accident, the man may begin to exhibit moderately dysfunctional behaviors. When his fourteen-year-old daughter needs to get to the airport on time, he might not be able to drive on that four-lane highway that is the sole route to the airport. Just the thought of such an endeavor might bring sweat to his palms. His heart may begin to race. Fear may tighten his chest. This distress may last until his daughter calls four other persons to get a ride to the airport. After this, the man may calm down and status quo may resume.

However, if this gentleman has a heart attack, then he truly is exhibiting impaired behavior. He may have developed a full-blown phobia, and the heart attack may be in addition to a panic attack. As such, he would have developed a mental disorder with potentially deadly consequences. The severity of complications that derives from the trauma of the accident now involved multiple areas of functioning, and the person is definitely considered impaired. Both the behaviors and the potential loss and grief issues must be addressed as soon as possible.

Sometimes the grief response also has varying internal and external manifestations. Christine is a woman who is quite willing to talk about her losses. This was true even though her losses were significant and some were traumatic. When asked about her grieving process she declared, "I've never cried." She didn't think it was right that she had not cried "after all these years." Christine was encouraged to talk more about her losses and her grief process. She really could go no further than to list them in somewhat of a cataloging way. When asked about how her life was going, she began to have more feeling. She said that she had "a short fuse," and that family had said that she had trashed her apartment and was threatening them. Everyone said she drank too much, but she didn't think she had a problem. When asked how long this had been going on, she stated that it had been two years. As it turned out, two years ago her mother had died and she was raped while walking in the park. This had been the precipitating grief reaction which set off the chain of events that left Christine in need of professional help.

Charting Severity of Grief Responses

Two charts demonstrate degrees of impairment in the feeling and in the transcendent or transpersonal area. In Table 3.2 the predominant feeling is anger. In Table 3.3 the predominant spiritual stressor is despair and hopelessness. While the charts are not meant to be ex-

TABLE 3.2. Severity of Grief Response
(Example of Response Continuum Regarding Feelings)

Normal	Mild Complication	Moderate Complication	Severe/dysfunctional Responses
Problems expressing feelings	Inability to express feelings	Absence of feelings	Rage Murder Suicide
		Pent-up or repressed feelings	Property destruction Arson
		Sleeping more	Bullying behavior Assaultive behavior
		Getting less done	Use of alcohol and drugs DWI
Stress	More Stress	Distress	Dysfunction/Impairment

TABLE 3.3. Severity of Grief Response
(Example of Response Continuum Regarding Spiritual Despair/Hope)

Normal	Mild Complication	Moderate Complicaton	Severe/Dysfunctional Responses
Prob-lems being hopeful	Inability to be very hopeful	Absence of hope	Despair Depression Anxiety Suicide
	Questions about God, higher power or pres-ence, and impor-tance of own spir-ituality	Pent-up or ex-pressed disap-pointment, anger with God	Unwillingness to for-give Blame Unrelenting guilt and shame Globalization of hope-lessness and helpless-ness or inflation of ego and grandiosity not otherwise evident in chemically based dis-order Paranoia about God, others, world's benevo-lence
	Lack of enthusi-asm or pleasure in relationships and interests	Avoidance of spir-itual practices that formerly enjoyed Stop going to church Anxiety about future	Aggressive behavior toward religion and those things connected with religion or spiritual practices Use of alcohol and drugs Counterculture activi-ties Amoral practices
Stress	More Stress	Distress	Dysfunction /Impair-ment

haustive, they do demonstrate possible movement from normal to dysfunctional grief.

The same kind of charts could be used for other possible complica-tions and impairment areas. These charts could be used as generic templates. Such is the case with the two mentioned previously. They could be available when completing the grief worksheet that was introduced in the previous chapter, and available in Appendix D. Since this kind of comparative process is helpful, a blank form titled Severity of Grief Response Impairment Flow Sheet is also provided in Appendix F.

The flow sheet would not be developed instead of the trajectory worksheet, but would allow a professional to go into specific problems descriptively and more thoroughly. For a total picture, information from individual flow sheets would be condensed and prioritized on a total treatment plan. In the situation charted for despair (Table 3.3), one therapist might focus on suicidal ideations; another might focus on forgiveness; and a third might focus on alcohol abuse. In the case involving anger (Table 3.2), one therapist might focus on behavioral rage outbursts; clergy might focus on development of trust and sharing feelings; and the law might focus on the DWI.

DYSFUNCTIONAL GRIEVING CRITERIA

Symptoms and Behavior That Can Indicate Dysfunctional Grieving

Although it is not always possible to accurately predict symptoms and behaviors that conclusively lead to dysfunctional grieving, it is possible to identify common clusters of behavior that, when present, increase the likelihood for dysfunctional grieving. These symptoms and behaviors can be used as criteria guidelines to assess the severity of dysfunction present or of potential concern. (For a brief chart of these symptoms and behaviors see Appendix G.)

Denial of Death or Loss

The denial of death, or the denial of any other significant life change (denial of divorce, financial condition, custody of children, etc.), when held for an extended time, can be seen as increasing the risk for grief to become dysfunctional. The key factors to discern are the pervasiveness of the denial, the insistence of denial after a reasonable time, and denial that persists when the grieving person is confronted with facts of death or loss.

Remember that denial is a normal, protective response to grief. When this protective response continues full force for a time, it can become a complication. But, when denial causes a person to engage in impaired responses that are harmful to self and others, it can be considered a part of a dysfunctional grief pattern.

For example, Edward had a normal and protective denial response to the loss of custody of his two children. Over and over again he declared, "This can't be happening!" This continued for days. Everyone was sympathetic at first, understanding this normal response. But the situation became more complicated when Edward began to wonder if it was that important to maintain ties with his children, and began to suggest that it wasn't worth the trouble. However, the day Edward went to his ex-wife's house and broke down the door, demanding that "things have not changed and they are not going to change," his ex-wife had no choice but to call the police. Weeks later, Edward talked about this, and the consequent restraining order. At this time even he admitted that he was in trouble, and had to face some facts about his divorce and his relationship to his children.

Aggressive, Violent, and Impulsive Behaviors

Two assumptions may be made in the consideration of violent and impulsive behavior as symptoms and behaviors that raise the risk factor for dysfunctional grieving responses. First, violent behavior is always evidence of dysfunction. Second, impulsive behavior must be assessed on the basis of harm or further impairment that results from the behavior. Suicidal behavior could also be considered impulsive and/or violent. At the same time, suicidal behavior may be part of a larger complicating factor, such as mental illness. Either way, these types of behaviors are dysfunctional, and may be related to complicated and dysfunctional grief.

However, violent and/or impulsive symptoms and behaviors that are dysfunctional grieving responses need to be assessed as relating directly to loss. Symptoms or behaviors that are not present prior to the loss, but occur in response to the loss, qualify as evidence of grief-related impairment. Those present prior to the loss may stem from previous losses, or be unrelated to grief. Thus, it is always crucial to make a careful study of the facts and circumstances before determining the cause or etiology of violent and impulsive behaviors. Loss often serves as a precipitating stressor that may bring about these kinds of responses.

Depression and Increasing Anxiety

Any form of depression or anxiety that interferes with normal, essential daily activity is evidence of a dysfunctional response. Persistent depression or pervasively increasing anxiety are diseases that may have chemical as well as situational roots. Grief, a situational root, can cause depression and anxiety. In fact, one of the concerns about significant, complicated, and severe grief responses is that an increased possibility exists for impairment to the point of developing a full-blown depression or anxiety disorder.

Eunice was a claims processor for an insurance company. The woman who shared the desk next to her died in a car accident when the car hit the abutment of a bridge and flipped over into the river below. Eunice was distraught about the loss of her friend, and after the funeral became aware that she felt incredible panic any time she drove over a bridge. Consequently, she refused to drive over any bridge, thus complicating her life. In Eunice's case, she needed to drive over bridges (particularly the one where her friend died) in order to get to work, visit her friends, and go to the grocery store. As time passed, she was able to work with her counselor to sort through her feelings about the loss of her friend, her fears about her own depression, and the prospect that her friend's death might have been a suicide. She was also able, through the prescription of anti-anxiety medication and cognitive-behavioral therapy, to reduce her fears about driving over bridges. Fortunately, the therapy was successful. However, Eunice's grief response demonstrates how grief can become dysfunctional very quickly, and severely limit the ability to live and enjoy life.

Extended Assignment of a Significant Loss As Cause for Current Difficulties

The assignment of a significant loss as cause for current difficulties may be due to intrapsychic impairment such as mechanisms of displacement or rationalization. As such, the response would be a defense. But, this kind of response may also be part of a larger difficulty with problem solving in general. Finally, this response may represent larger cognitive challenges. In truth, this kind of response is really a symptom statement that requires further investigation.

Since in some cases a current difficulty can directly relate to a loss, or multiple losses, it is crucial to gather enough data to determine the nature and extent of the hypothesized connection. However, when further exploration does not yield understandable connections with current difficulties, other sources must be considered. Of course, it may still be the case that displacement or rationalization may be symptoms of previously unfinished or dysfunctional grieving.

In Chet's case, he never seemed to finish what he started. However, his colleagues didn't know this was a lifelong habit. During a particularly frustrating period at work he would say that he just couldn't concentrate because he was thinking of his father. Or he would say, "I still miss my father." Or, he would launch into stories of how his father, who was in the same profession, used to handle similar things. After such a story, he would conclude that he guessed he learned how to do things the old-fashioned way as his father did before him. This all went according to Chet's plan, because people would back off, thinking that he was still acutely grieving the death of his father. They would let his lack of productivity slip by.

However, one day Chet got a new partner who was younger and more energetic. It only took the new partner several months of hearing Chet's reasoning for his lack of productivity before he realized that something was wrong. The partner confronted Chet. The clue for him was that Chet showed no other signs of grief. In fact, Chet never seemed to think of his father unless he was explaining why he wasn't getting things done. To make matters worse, everyone discovered that Chet's father had died a very long time ago. Chet confessed that he had the problem of not finishing what he started for as long as he could remember. Everyone agreed that enough was enough, and that Chet needed help. They were no longer going to let him off the hook.

Lingering Spiritual Distress or Despair

Invariably, existential bitterness, loss of trust, loss of faith, and loss of hope are symptoms of grief that become complicating factors and can lead to dysfunctional behaviors. The longer these responses linger, the greater the chance of significant impairment and disease. Usually the loss must be significant, traumatic, and part of a group of significant losses for these responses to cause lasting impairment. As a safety precaution, it is extremely important to take an extensive loss history when these symptoms are present. It may even be wise to go back through several generations to discover what might have been happening in the extended family, with ancestors, and even in the broader culture. Spiritual distress or despair is perceived as an existential threat that often makes the larger world seem unfriendly and malevolent. Dysfunction can present itself on a continuum that may include unstable relationships, unproductive attempts to achieve personal and professional goals, and antisocial behaviors.

Extended Withdrawal from Formerly Comforting Relationships

Here the impairment is one of isolation and withdrawal as a grief response. One young woman declared, after several relationships with boyfriends that left her grieving and hurt, "I'm going to stay single." This is a normal grieving response. However, it was stated after an overdose that nearly resulted in death. In many cases, a pervasive and extended withdrawal from relationships is a symptom of depression or an anxiety.

Harmful Practices

Most people go through a normal process of eating more or less after a loss. Some temporarily need to take a mild sedative, anti-depressant, or anxiety medication. It is equally common to experience irritability and have trouble getting work done. Normally these changes are transient and have mild or moderate consequences that go away as the grief process continues.

However, the following harmful practices may indicate dysfunctional grieving:

- Reliance on or abuse of drugs and alcohol or addictive substances, such as use of tobacco-related products or high intake of caffeine-related substances
- Health-threatening overeating or undereating
- Reliance on or noncompliance with medications
- Excessive exercise or extreme lethargy over time

These harmful practices may indicate dysfunctional grieving. They may also be due to illnesses or prior difficulties. To determine if a practice is harmful, a careful history and assessment is necessary. Questions of when the behavior began and the circumstances that surround the behavior will help to determine whether these changes are grief related. However, experience dictates that some loss, or fear of loss, is almost always involved when these four practices shift dramatically. Still, caution is required, since many behaviors are harmful, but they are not equally harmful. Often, successful treatment results from addressing the most harmful behaviors first, and putting others temporarily on a "to do list."

Sandra was referred for therapy after being raped. Further history revealed sexual abuse over an extended time. In addition to these traumas, Sandra had a history of several instances trying to injure herself through extremely harmful behaviors. However, she arrived for therapy with a happy smile, declaring that everything was fine and that she didn't need therapy. Since she was in blatant denial and experiencing what is often called "a flight to health" it did not make sense to ignore these symptoms.

Fortunately, Sandra had been court ordered to get treatment, since she was the mother of small children and drugs were involved. Yet, it took a long time to get an extended loss history, and an even longer time to help her link her grieving experiences to the high-risk, harmful behaviors that followed. Her situation was more manageable because she was an in-patient without access to drugs, and her children were being well cared for by other family members.

Dependency

Dependency after a significant loss is common, and is usually a transient symptom. Sometimes, this response is part of a person's personality and lifestyle prior to the loss, and becomes more intense as a result of the loss. This can be true when dependent people lose a relationship that helped them function, or was intimately tied up in their identity.

On the other hand, some are not dependent prior to a significant loss but become more and more dependent. Thus, their dependency can be clearly related to the loss and complications during the grief process. This kind of dependency can be particularly frightening, because the person is not accustomed to being dependent. A dependent person is not so concerned about being dependent, but is afraid of being independent. The difference is significant when considering approach and treatment.

Maureen had a dependent personality and lived a dependent lifestyle most of her life. After her husband of fifty-two years died, she went to live with her daughter and son-in-law. Since she had been very dependent on her husband for many years, she naturally transferred this dependence to her daughter. However, things did not go smoothly and everyone was soon highly stressed.

Maureen was angry that her daughter would not give up her job and stay home to take care of her. Her daughter was convinced that she could easily do many of these things for herself. Needless to say, Maureen got clingy and tried to get her daughter to quit her job. She did her best to make her daughter feel obligated to do this, for this was the way her "father would have wanted it."

It only took a few months for the daughter and son-in-law to feel driven to the edge of divorce by Maureen's demands. Thus, after one particularly awful bout, the daughter called her brother, and insisted that Maureen come and stay with him and his family. However, the brother feared his mother's dependency also, and decided that this only be a temporary arrangement.

At the son's house things were no better. Both adults worked and Maureen was once again left at home. She was so furious that she agreed to take the first opening in a nursing home that had an assisted living unit. She didn't care what the cost. After all, her third child who lived a thousand miles away was in charge of the finances and ensuring that her needs were met. One week later, Maureen moved into an assisted living unit where she received some of the attention she craved, and (to her dismay) experienced some appropriate limit setting by the staff. Maureen moved from assisted living to a health care unit at a young age, much earlier than her age and capabilities would warrant. But a lifelong habit and personality deficit was a constant challenge that complicated everyone's grief, blocked internal grief processing, and hindered relationships within the family.

Risk Taking

Frequently, complicated and dysfunctional grieving patterns involve varying degrees of risk taking that are not part of a person's former personality profile. This risk taking may involve a lack of attention and caution that was formerly used in everyday life. It also can involve putting oneself in danger just to test the life consequences. Problematic risks often occur in activities, relationships, and general testing or disregard for health and safety. Risks that can be part of the dysfunctional grieving pattern include the following:

- Lack of self-care
- Driving excessively fast
- Road rage
- Binge drinking/drugging
- Breaking the law
- Carelessness in using machinery
- Extramarital affairs

Lingering Sense of General Foreboding

A pervasive sense of foreboding is a common thought and feeling present in traumatic losses. This is particularly true when these losses have had horrible consequences in one's life. In some cases, there is reason for the foreboding and this can complicate grief and may cause dysfunctional responses. For example, a person who has remarried and becomes aware of similar patterns of escalating violence may have reason to be concerned. In other cases, the foreboding surrounds future losses that appear to have no rational basis. The risk here is for impairment in health and in general functioning on all levels. A pervasive sense of doom hanging over a person's future indicates a need for appropriate and timely intervention.

INDIVIDUALS WHO ARE PARTICULARLY AT RISK

People who are particularly at risk for dysfunctional grieving are those who have complications such as described in Chapter 2. From a clinical and pastoral perspective, individuals who are particularly at risk for dysfunctional grief experience loss as a threat to inner, relational, and environmental stability and well-being.

Individuals with Vulnerability to Stress

Some professionals consider biological vulnerability and environmental stress to be handmaidens to consequent mental disorders. Strictly speaking, any loss is a stressor. For this reason, people who are vulnerable to stress may have complications that make their grief more prone to dysfunctional symptoms and behavior. At the same time, people who have had no previous difficulty with grieving may find themselves particularly vulnerable at times. Therefore, it is best to consider a person who is currently vulnerable at risk for impaired symptoms and behaviors.

Individuals with Concurrent Mental Disorders Including Organic Injuries

People with mental disorders, including organic injuries, are at risk for complicated and dysfunctional grieving. However, this does not mean their losses will always lead to dysfunctional responses. In general, though, those who have a concurrent mental disorder, or a consequent disorder, will have some impairment in capacity to move through the stages of grief.

Individuals with Ambivalent Values and Beliefs

In this instance a hypothesis is being offered that counterculture values and beliefs can put a person at risk for dysfunctional grieving. Certainly such beliefs can be complicating factors. However, this hypothesis is drawn from experience more than from research, yet it has been shown that beliefs and values do effect functioning (see Koenig, 1997).

Esther wanted to die. She was eighty-nine and had lost her spouse a dozen years ago. Her hearing and eyesight were poor. Although family support was excellent, her life had changed as she aged. To a certain degree, she had never been independent and had struggled with mild depression and anxiety. For both of these disorders she had taken mild doses of medication and her deceased spouse had waited on her hand and foot. In their retirement years she didn't even walk to the bathroom by herself. Still, she did fairly well. By the time she was eighty-nine she began to make sure that everyone was crystal clear regarding her funeral arrangements. In fact she was overcontrolling, as usual, about this matter. In addition, she began to talk more about her husband and her desire to be with him. She believed in eternal life, including the faith that she would see loved ones who had passed on before. Esther's history of early grief experiences was complicated, and she was somewhat dysfunctional emotionally for much of her life. However, at the age of eighty-nine her beliefs seemed quite normal and she no longer evidenced dysfunction. In fact, just the opposite was true. Esther had recovered and her faith had been one important aspect of that recovery.

In Tim's case, his lack of beliefs and ever-shifting values put him at risk for dysfunctional grieving. He did not believe in God or a higher power. He had been in trouble with the law since he was a teen and had relied on alcohol and drugs to ease his pain. As a teen he was given the diagnosis of oppositional-defiant disorder and he was somewhat proud of it. Tim knew he was on his own, and often declared that he just didn't care what society or anyone had to say about his life. However, through all this, Tim had a mother who loved him. When she died, he was truly alone and was found late one night nearly dead from a self-inflicted gunshot wound. Apparently, Tim's mother had been the one person he had counted on in life.

Individuals with Multiple and Traumatic Losses

People with multiple and traumatic losses are at risk for complicated and dysfunctional grieving responses. Multiple grief experiences challenge an already grieving person's capacity to recover from one loss before the next one occurs. Traumatic losses that come from horrible events often burn equally horrendous and unfathomable memories and questions into the mind. In the case of traumatic losses, the risk exists for developing a full-blown post-traumatic stress disorder.

Individuals Whose Support System Is Severely Challenged or Impaired

Frequently, the drastic change of a support system due to a loss causes complications to the grieving process. When these supports helped with daily functioning and emotional stability, the risk for dysfunction increases.

Janice was a young adult when she had a car accident. She had to relearn almost all activities of daily living. However, she was highly motivated and surprised everyone by her comeback. This comeback seemed miraculous until her father died.

Her father's death left her without much stability. It was difficult for her to process his death. She did not live close to her father, but she relied on an idealized image of him that was partially fulfilled when she visited him. Even though she was close to her mother, she intensely missed her father. Her mother was a hard worker who had to support the family and maintain some sense of order. At times, Janice thought that the person who should have been a mom was now just a bit critical and distant emotionally. For her mom's part, she just didn't have the time to spend with Janice and wished that things were otherwise.

Time was often a blur to Janice. She spent much of her time at home and had few friends. The few friends that she retained from her younger years were growing older and getting jobs, and sometimes starting families. Years later, Janice overdosed on medication. She survived the incident and was referred for grief therapy. Her thoughts before the overdose were that she wanted to be with her dad.

Janice was a hard worker and her mother considered the overdose a wake-up call. Both engaged in individual and family therapy, learning coping skills, communication skills, and the need to extend the support resources for their family. Their joint and separate grief work brought them closer together than ever before.

STRATEGIES FOR CHALLENGING
DYSFUNCTIONAL BEHAVIOR

Severely dysfunctional grief must be addressed as soon as possible for the well-being of the individual, and those who relate to him or her. When the individual exhibits even moderately dysfunctional behavior, there may also be a need to set limits and to facilitate behavioral change. Of particular concern is a need to prevent challenging behaviors from escalating into more damaging responses.

For helpers who are used to a softer or gentler approach, confronting behaviors can be a challenging part of working with dysfunctional grief. In the first place, stopping behaviors is not easy. Second, the helper is often in a position that he or she would not prefer to be in as helper. This is particularly true of therapists and clergy who prefer to present themselves as empathic and caring. In some cases, the person being challenged may exhibit increased negative behaviors that may be targeted at the helper. Plus, there is the risk that the person will go elsewhere for help, or choose to receive no help at all.

As a rule, some approaches work better than others. The choice of which approach to use must always be a matter of what will work best, has the least negative effect, and will fit the person, the helper, and the relationship.

Unhelpful Approaches

Some approaches that are often not successful:

- Drawing on external power or authority, including the helper's, someone else's, or transcendent sources. Usually this just becomes one more powerful force taking something else away.
- Threatening with negative consequences, particularly if one does not have the power to enforce the threat. This approach can escalate behavior. In some cases, the person may feel that challenging threats must be treated with equal power so that some control can be restored.
- Use of seductive methods, such as manipulation, even when disguised as professionally grounded. Even attempts to coddle or distract may be perceived as condescending and therefore resented.
- Forcing or pushing values and choices that are not intrinsically of value to the individual. Often people are looking for better choices than the ones they are using, but haven't been successful so far. When choices are presented that seem foreign to their lifestyle, they feel coerced or confused. They feel violated when required to be other than they are.

- Any response that may indicate that the helper doesn't care and that everything depends upon the individual. This may be perceived as abandonment and becomes another loss. It also may be experienced as a hostile approach, which it is.

More Helpful Approaches

Some helpful approaches include the following:

- Focus on values—sorting and sifting through various values that may be considered
- Acknowledge that adult thinking may be different from earlier, younger, thinking
- Reframe the desire to be good, do the best one can, be a caring person
- Just say "stop"—in cases of safety and harm to self and others
- Provide choices—even better, help the person consider choices
- Focus on free will and choice, with acknowledgment that the individual may consider the current approach worth the problems and consequences that follow
- Share personal/professional opinion, having stated that this is the source of what is being shared
- Encourage others (if family or group work) to share their experiences with the situation
- Explain essential action in a nonthreatening manner, with caring tone and with clarity. Do not say more than necessary and express willingness to check back with the person, or convey that the relationship is still intact even though the negative behavior must stop.
- Brainstorm other approaches and behavioral responses
- Explore with the person possible causes for the behavior
- Engage a second opinion
- Refer to a psychiatrist or primary care provider to rule out possibilities for other explanations for behaviors
- Ask how current behavior and responses are working for the individual. Often they are not working well. A discussion could then follow about what might work better given the person's desire and needs.

Use of Grief Trajectory Worksheet
for Dysfunctional Grieving

In the Grief Trajectory Worksheet discussed in Chapter 2, an obstacle or problem can be defined as complication or as dysfunction. Otherwise, the same form can be used for complicated as for dysfunctional grief. If the grief is assessed as dysfunctional, it would make sense for complications to be listed separately from dysfunction (see Appendix D). Steps to completing this worksheet for dysfunctional grieving are as follows:

1. Complete Grief Trajectory Worksheet.
2. Review history of functioning and include in loss history if it is not already there.
3. List dysfunctional behaviors in the column marked "obstacles" (problems). Be sure to describe the dysfunctional behavior.
4. Place a large X on Grief Trajectory Template to indicate stage(s) that may be causing the dysfunction.
5. Summarize dysfunctional symptoms and behaviors and place a risk assessment next to the list. Use a scale of 0 (none) to 5 (high) to determine degree of risk to self or to others.

SUMMARY

Some professionals find it easy to listen to a grief story and translate the information in terms of function and impairment. Others may resist using clinical or health care language. If one resists the use of clinical language, one must still find a way to assess, diagnose, and refer people whose grief has become dysfunctional. Likewise, if one resists the use of descriptive language for spiritual processes, or even the inclusion of spiritual assessment, one must still find a way to assess, diagnose and refer people whose grief has become spiritually dysfunctional. In any case, dysfunctional grief must always receive timely and appropriate treatment to prevent great risk to health and life.

Chapter 4

The Spiritual Side of Grief and Loss

As we name more accurately the outline of our own spirit, we begin to look for that same spirit in those we meet. Slowly we may begin to feel less alone and more part of a family of children, all of whom hurt, all of whom ache for love.

Muller, 1993, p. 163

It was midmorning when Fred asked if he could come into the office and talk. He sat down and stretched out his legs so that his feet could rest on the table in front of him. He sat there quietly for some time. After a while I asked him how he was doing. He looked at me rather quizzically and said, "Physically, I am doing well." Then he took a shallow breath, paused, and declared, "But spiritually I'm not doing so well." He spoke of the divorce proceedings that had just been completed; of separation from his young child; of alcoholism; and of being broke. He also said he had terminal cancer.

Fred said he believed in God. While growing up he attended church, but he didn't think he had to go to church in order to be good. He added that he hadn't prayed in a long time. Then, as the conversation continued, he began to wonder about the Hindu faith and coming back as a fish. He thought this would befit his current life. He continued to talk about the idea of reincarnation. Finally, he concluded, "I have made many mistakes, and I'm going to meet God soon, so I had better take that into consideration." He finished with the AA motto, "Right now I'm just taking one day at a time." He stood up. His head drooped just a little as he said, "Thank you," and left.

DEFINITION OF SPIRITUALITY

In a recent report, published by the Fetzer Institute, the following definition of spirituality was adapted for use in research on the effects of spirituality and religion on mental and physical health.

> Spirituality is concerned with the transcendent, addressing ultimate questions about life's meaning, with the assumption that there is more to life than what we see or fully understand. Spirituality can call us beyond self to concern and compassion for others. (Fetzer Institute, 1999, p. 2)

This report grouped spirituality and religiousness under one term. To quote the working group that developed this instrument for the measurement of religiousness/spirituality,

> While religions aim to foster and nourish the spiritual life, and spirituality is often a salient aspect of religious participation, it is possible to adopt the outward forms of religious worship and doctrine without having a strong relationship to the transcendent. (Fetzer Institute, 1999, p. 2)

For the purposes of this book, spirituality has a broader definition than the one adopted by the National Institute on Aging Working Group. This interpretation does not limit spirituality to a transcendent function, or relationship, nor does it limit religion to outward doctrine and practices. Given the diversity of human experience, a broader definition will more accurately represent life experience, in general, and grief, in particular. The following definition of spirituality offers this broader context:

> Spirituality is that which provides meaning, purpose, and connection for an individual, a group of individuals, a community, and/or a culture.

Thus, spirituality has to do with those experiences that relate to all levels of existence. These levels of experience can be visualized as moving from the most individualized internal functions of the human spirit, through human relationships and beyond, to forces that connect to, and perhaps transcend, human experience and understanding.

This progression is shown in Boxes 4.1 and 4.2. Although the experiences of integrated spiritual relationship are listed vertically in these figures, there is no presumption that spirituality is confined to such restricted order.

Transcendent and transpersonal spirituality points to the spiritual dimension that provides connectedness within personal, transpersonal, and transcendent spheres. Dynamically, the energy within this level is always working toward relationship and connection between relational components. Thus, at the transcendent/transpersonal level of spiritual experience, spiritual connectedness is the active destination of all experience. Hence the nouns, outreach and connection, are appropriate terms for provisions of the transcendent/transpersonal spirit. This means that an initial inquiry into issues of loss is always, among other things, a spiritual inquiry into the spirit of connection and disconnection.

At the intimate, or in-reach, level of spiritual experience, spirit is not so much a destination as it is representative of the interior actions that lead toward the destination of outreach and promote connection. Many actions promote spirit, but the components listed above are especially essential to recovery. Impairment in the efforts of any of

---

BOX 4.1. *Transcendent/Transpersonal Spirituality* or Outreach

> Higher spirit/power/God/Goddesses
> Spirit of creation
> Cultural spirit
> Communal spirit
> Individual spirit

BOX 4.2. *Intimate Spirituality* or In-Reach

Spirit of being and believing
Spirit of creating and growing
Spirit of acting and generating
Spirit of witnessing and lighting
    (as in process of enlightenment)

these actions leave one spiritually disconnected (in troubled or impaired relationship).

Finally, even though spirituality has to do with the levels of experience listed previously, it is not confined to these two levels. For, spirit has its own creative and generative functions that aim toward integration and connection. Therefore, spirit, or the spiritual dimension, is connected to, but autonomous from, other biopsychosocial and emotional dimensions.

Outreach or in-reach spiritual activity can be enhanced through any and all experiences. As such, appropriate interventions provided during the grief process can also enhance spiritual activity. Conversely, outreach and in-reach experiences can also become impaired by unhelpful interventions. Even so, the burden is not completely on the grieving person, or on the helper. Healing and recovery can happen out of its own purpose, sense of meaning, and intrinsic striving for connection. Thus transcendent and transpersonal functions often contribute autonomously to religious and humanistic spirituality.

RELIGIOUS SPIRITUALITY

Religious spirituality also addresses all of the experiences of spirituality that are listed in Boxes 4.1 and 4.2. In addition, religious spirituality aims to create order and ritual out of diverse spiritual experiences, thus providing meaning, companioning, and spirit to relationships. In this sense, religion is a system for holding all aspects of spirituality in tension with one another in a creative and positive way. At its best, it does so through the use of all of the senses and dimensions of human functioning.

Religious/spiritual dogma (or teachings) speaks to the mind, and to the search for meaning, purpose, and connection. Practices (such as worship, sacraments, rituals, prayers, charity, social action, and witness) speak to forms and functions that help individuals, communities, and cultures remain spiritually focused. These practices also help people be connected and spiritually interactive. Interior associations, connections, and changes promoted by religious spirituality also speak to the movement of spirit and therefore to spirituality. In this sense, religious spirituality is not just church, synagogue, world religion, or denomination. Rather, religious spirituality refers to any system of spiritual integration that relies on the continuum of intimate and transcendent levels of spirituality, for the purpose of integration and wholeness. Thus, paganism, new age systems, and cults can be considered forms of religious spirituality.

The strength of religious spirituality is the spirit of connection over time, in all circumstances, and at all levels of experience. In *Life Together,* originally written in 1938, pastor Dietrich Bonhoeffer speaks of the effects of communal spirituality, even when individuals are separated from community. According to Bonhoeffer,

> It is by the grace of God that a congregation is permitted to gather visibly to share in God's Word and sacrament. Not all Christians receive this blessing. The imprisoned, the sick, the scattered lonely, the proclaimers of the Gospel in heathen lands stand alone. They know that visible fellowship is a blessing. . . . But they remain alone in far countries, a scattered seed according to God's will. Yet what is denied them as an actual experience they seize upon more fervently in faith. (Bonhoeffer, 1954, pp. 18-19)

It is probably impossible to be religiously spiritual externally without some inner spiritual activity, although the two may not be well integrated. So, too, is it not possible to be interiorly spiritual without external manifestations? Although people often find it wise to restrict some spiritual practice expressions in certain situations.

However, the term religious spirituality has been so restricted by cultural and social custom, for practical purposes, it is not sufficiently broad enough to encompass all experiences of spirituality. Some individuals, communities, and cultures have not found meaning, purpose, and connection through these spiritual expressions. For these people, spirituality is a private internal expression that does not include transcendent connections, and may not include communal, or cultural, connections either. Since this is true, there are times when it would be appropriate to just use the term spirituality, and include religious spirituality under the broader umbrella of spirituality. However, one could not reverse the process and use religious spirituality as the umbrella for all spirituality. So, religious spirituality (or religiousness/spirituality) is reserved for occasions when the transcendent or transpersonal function is included in an orderly manner that can be replicated and provide meaning for those who are so connected.

SPIRITUALITY AND WELLNESS

Since mind, body, and spirit are interconnected, they can only be separated for the purpose of reflection, communication, and to set forth a professional scope of practice that provides for the use and limitation of certain interventions. Yet, separation for any of these purposes is not easy. Although the interconnectedness of all things is a well-known fact in today's postmodern world, the subtleties of this connection continue to need further exploration.

Thus, some researchers exhibit an ever-growing desire to continue to explore the spirit part of the mind, body, and spirit triad. The focus of these researchers has been on the impact of spiritual beliefs and practices on health and wellness. In addition to identifying the mechanisms by which spirituality in general affects human functioning, research has also been conducted on the positive outcomes gained as the direct result of certain spiritual practices, such as prayer (see Dossey, 1993).

Although this book does not focus on the specifics of this research, studies have been conducted that connect specific positive attitudes and spiritual practices with improved health and wellness. For example, regular attendance at church and prayer (White and MacDougall, 2001, pp. 3-9) has been shown to promote health and healing. For more information on current research, the reader is encouraged to refer to the works of Koenig (1997), Benson (1996) and Dossey (1993).

In general, spirituality promotes wellness when it provides meaning, purpose, and connection through the selection and use of meaningful thoughts, feelings, and practices. In times of health and well-being, life is meaningful, purposeful, and a sense of connectedness prevails. During these times, the world is considered benevolent. There is an overall existential experience of more gain than loss. Thus, normal functioning during periods with minimum loss includes positive levels of spiritual experiences, and interior activity that promotes connection. By analyzing these levels of spiritual experience, the clinician can find clues to the development of complicated and dysfunctional grief responses.

Spiritual Well-Being As Living in the Garden of Eden

An interesting example of a natural state of spiritual well-being is found in the ancient scripture of Genesis (1: 1-31). Here we find in story form a description of how God created everything and upon reflection, declared it good. Delightfully, the first integrated spiritual state provided for humans occurred as the culmination of creation. This integrated spiritual state is described contextually as living in "the Garden of Eden." This is an early metaphor, or spiritual fact. We are born into a time of potential gain and abundance. We are created with the spiritual intention to live and grow in a state of contented relationship.

The Garden of Eden is a good place. The experience of it is part of each person's inheritance and destination. Thus, we are forever in search of recovering this place. Some call it calm. Some call it peace. Some call it serenity. For, apparently, there is not much hard work during these contented times of gain, when we are spiritually in the gardens of our life. At these times, our actions are very appropriate. Life comes together easily. But this garden, like every other garden, is alive and has its seasons. Later on, the story will deal with the loss that occurs even in beautiful gardens. The experience of these seasons is also our inheritance.

From our losses we will learn that even in the midst of gain, seeds of change occur, together with another natural process, loss. When the consequences of these seeds of change come to light, then spiritual distress manifests. This necessitates grief work, the hard toiling into new, unexplored areas. The good news is that all of us have times of spiritual wellness and we draw from these experiences in times of spiritual distress.

SPIRITUAL ACTIVITY

Spirituality provides the daily capacity to ACT on our own behalf and in connection with others. Spiritual acts are connected to mind and body, and have unique life-promoting functions that are essential to living well. Spiritual actions have their own ways of acknowledging reality, of containing thoughts and feelings, and of promoting meaning. Just as the mind generates its own thoughts and feelings, and the body generates its own responses and actions, so too can the spiritual life generate meaning and action. Thus, spiritual acts acknowledge reality (including transcendent and transpersonal realities), contain thoughts and feelings, and open a space for action (through trust or faith). This, then, is the gift of spirituality—the capacity to act.

The Capacity to ACT

A acknowledge reality
At multiple levels and complexities perhaps including
the reality of a transcendent or higher power

C contain thoughts and feelings
That can be varied and unstable and wonder about the thoughts
and feelings of others and possibly the divine other

T trust process and respond accordingly
Open space for faith/trust and action

Health and Wellness Promoting Actions of Spirit

Some of the spiritual processes that constitute the activity of the spirit and its work toward promoting health and wellness are found in the following list. The list is not exhaustive but is suggestive of how spiritual activity promotes health and wellness:

- Spiritual activity generates motivation and initiative.
- Spiritual activity comes from the heart and values relationship.
- Spiritual activity increases one's capacity to respond, endure, and stay the course during the good and the challenging times.
- Spiritual activity remembers and contributes a larger perspective.
- Spiritual activity creates a container for holding feelings and anchoring particularly painful ones such as anxiety, sorrow, and anger.
- Spiritual activity is a carrier of meaning, rationale or purpose, and feedback.
- Spiritual activity comes as guidance and wise counsel.
- Spiritual activity leads to behavior and creatively responds to rituals of past, present, and future.
- Spiritual activity brings comfort and compassion.
- Spiritual activity is future oriented and therefore has a challenging edge.
- Spiritual activity uplifts ethical conversation.

- Spiritual activity is carried on the energy of character-based attributes.
- Spiritual activity tends toward altruism while promoting individual needs.
- Spiritual activity has as its aim instrumental healing and change and is outcome oriented.

THE SPIRITUAL COMPONENT OF GRIEF WORK

The primary function of spirit, and of spiritual activity during grief, is to make sense of loss and address the changed relational reality. After a significant loss, this intrinsic striving for renewal, or reconnection, is accomplished through the grieving process. To this end, the spiritual dimension joins mind and body as respondent and as active partner in the cocreation of a new reality. Together, these three dimensions strive to relate to what is happening, and to gain equilibrium.

The spiritual component does its part by acting as resource for finding meaning from loss. This meaning-making process is used as a connecter to other mind and body processes that are also at work. Understanding spiritual activities as being integral to internal dialogical processes, helps in understanding the grief work process and the movement toward recovery. Recovery in this sense occurs when a new understanding, or internal/relational connectedness, is reached that is satisfactory to mind, body, and spirit.

Positive Effects of Spirituality on Grieving

During normal grief, an individual's spirituality is usually supportive of the grieving process. For during grief, most of the actions of spirit are activated with the intention of moving toward healing and recovery. Of course, some actions are more evident at one stage than others. This spiritual activation makes sense, as meaning, purpose, and connection are essential to each stage of recovery.

However, even though the actions of spirit are normally health promoting and strive toward integration, sometimes a person will access spiritual resources in negative ways. On these occasions, grief can be said to have become spiritually complicated, and the grief process may become dysfunctional. It is not spirit that is dysfunctional, but a person's inner and outer expressions of spirituality.

Spiritual Stressors, Distress, and Disease

Because an individual's experience of spirituality can become complicated and even impaired, the negative consequences of spiritual distress are just as potentially risky as negative consequences of the functions of mind and body. This is so because all significant losses bring experiences of disconnection that temporarily challenge meaning, purpose, and connection. When disconnection is not restored in a timely manner, distress, dysfunction, and disease can develop.

Distressed and diseased spirituality impairs the daily capacity to act on one's own behalf and in connection with others. In the case of spiritual distress, dysfunction, and disease the actions of personal spirit RESIST rather than ACT.

Spiritual Distress – An Urge to RESIST

R resist reality of mind, body, and spiritual matters
E employ distorted thinking
S sense feelings that are predominantly negative
I increase intensity of chaotic processes that are hard to contain become rigid and narrow
S stuck in distrust
T tend toward chaotic and destructive actions

Spiritual distress and dysfunction mean that the individual spirit is not functioning well and is in need of appropriate treatment. However, it does not necessarily mean that the ultimate source of spirit has been impaired or diminished in capacity. Nor does spiritual distress imply that the essence and activity of intimate spirit, and the essence and activity of transcendent/transpersonal functions, are not striving to achieve healing and recovery.

Lisa experienced spiritual distress as she grieved Barry's impending death. Barry was dying of cancer. He went through a gradual decline in health and increasingly remained in bed. Comfort measures were provided. These measures worked fairly well, but occasionally he was in pain. During his last days, family and friends visited him to say good-bye. Lisa, a longtime friend, was visiting him during his last hour. She had struggled hard about making the decision to visit Barry, but ultimately she felt good about doing so. While the hospice nurse was attending to Barry's body, Lisa lingered in the other room with tears flowing gently down her cheeks.

Upon seeing Lisa's tears, another friend rushed up to Lisa to assure her that Barry was OK. He would be buried and when Jesus came again he would likely be raised up to heaven. Meanwhile it was just his body in the grave.

Even though the friend was trying to be helpful, Lisa burst into even greater sobs. She hadn't thought of Barry lying, for who knows how long, in the ground. She had pictured his spirit as ascending at the moment of death right up to heaven. She believed that he would immediately be with God. This belief had strengthened her and gave her courage during the past hour. Now, who knows what would happen! Maybe when Jesus came again, he wouldn't even recognize Barry. Maybe Barry wouldn't be one of the chosen ones. Maybe he would stay in the ground forever.

As the days went by, Lisa couldn't shake her feelings of sadness and despair. She found herself sinking farther and farther into the pits of doubt and distrust. She stopped attending church. She couldn't face looking at the crucifix. She could no longer take the Eucharist with confidence. She told no one. After all, whom would she tell? Her family was staunchly Catholic and would just say this was silly.

Other changes began to take place. Lisa became sullen and withdrawn at work. She got up later and later, and began to call in sick frequently. When spring came she did not work in her garden. When confronted with the changes, she declared, "What's the use?"

Because spirit's natural state is one of active connection, and distress of the spirit is demonstrated in resistance, grief can become quite complicated. One of the most difficult things to accept, after a significant loss, is the fact that loss is part of the essence of reality. Thus, grief is like day and night; it comes and goes without our input.

Some people have tried to understand this distressing fact of creation. The first experience of loss and grief found in sacred scripture was mentioned earlier in the brief reference to the Garden of Eden. The same story, previously told in the context of religious spirituality, can also be told in the spirit of general spirituality with a case for complicated grief as also being a part of reality.

Creation's Tale Revisited:
And Then There Was Complicated Grief

One eternal morning, the only power that could create decided to make a change. Surrounded by oneness, the power decided to create two. So it happened that the second was mighty dark and deep. This was not change enough, so a powerful light was added to the mix. Then it really became clear that there were all kinds of complexity.

But power was not intimidated by complexity. Instead, power embraced it and time was also thrown into the mix, bringing with it more ways to mark change and remember complexity. So it was that time became filled with everything. Needless to say everything created quite a commotion. One never could tell what everything was up to or even where it was headed.

All this change was good, and power was quite energized by it. In fact, everything was growing so complex that power decided to become more at one with all this complexity. So, it contributed not just from its powerful self, but out of a part of itself, something new was born. Some say the newness was gender, but that didn't really make sense, for power had no gender. Whatever it was, it came forth as something new, and it, too, was filled with so much power that it felt empowered. Meantime, the only power that could create took a break and reveled in all the intricacies of complexity.

However, it happened that complexity was used to change and could not stop changing, even if it wanted to do so. Plus, power had grown used to action and diversity, and yearned for more, and, as change would have it, power had also grown more reflective during the break and began to develop a desire for more empowered ones. So, the created and empowered one became two, but not the same two.

By now, nothing could stop change. Feelings began to get more complex and started to operate on their own. In truth, the only power that could create tried to stop change, and to limit complexity, by setting limits on the empowered ones. But this could not happen, for now things were the way they were. So complexity became known as life. Creation was creation. Plus, the empowered two were partnered so that they too could grow and create their own complexity.

So it was that there became a name for everything, and so much complexity that everything couldn't be controlled. This was when grief came into the picture. Born of change, remembered in time, developed out of powerful feelings, and nurtured by reflection, the seeds of grief were treasured and empowered to manage diversity, complexity, and even change, which seemed to have become so complex that everything was now quite challenging.

Sometime later, an empowered one who felt grief, and was overwhelmed by everything, began to wonder why grief was even part of life. Some blamed gender and others blamed everything they could. But only the power to create knew what had really happened. Only the power to create knew for sure why grief was intended to be a part of life right from the beginning. For power remembered the day that grief was born. It was born the day after complexity, when change set everything in motion. Thus, power remembered its creative thought. "Good grief," it had reflected, "it's going to be hard work from here on dealing with all this change." So it was that grief was born as a gift especially suited to dealing with change and complexity.

EXPERIENCES OF SPIRITUALLY BASED GRIEF COMPLICATIONS

Certain spiritually based issues tend to be activated in times of grief and have the tendency to develop into complications. Although not exhaustive, the list of issues includes the following:

    Presence and abandonment
    Righteousness and bad things happening
    Tests and challenges
    Suffering, creation, and deliverance
    Capacity of God/Higher Power and use of miracles
    Times when it may be too much to bear
    Commandment to forgive
    Guilt
    Spirituality versus science

These complications come from spirituality bumping into other realities such as mind and body, social and cultural wisdom, and religious spiritual traditions. Particularly complicated are the losses that seem to happen for no reason, or no good reason! When there is no good reason for a loss it seems senseless. When a reason for loss such as lung disease (as a result of smoking three packs of cigarettes a day) is apparent, then spirit is distressed, but in reality, understands the loss.

Some losses seem to be beyond the ordinary. These losses cause spiritual work to be all the more difficult. When these losses occur, spiritual questions are often formulated in efforts to cope.

> Why does a parent abandon a child?
> Why does a good person suffer with illness and pain?
> Why does God give some people too much to bear?
> Why doesn't prayer work or miracles happen for me?
> Why wasn't I there for him or her?
> Does God even care?

When these questions are asked they are not abstract questions, but rather are painful human grief concerns and should be treated accordingly.

A small part of each spiritually based concern is provided in the following vignette. This format retains the power of the concern, while providing a temporary image and context for the dilemma. The healing power found in these examples is due to the use of a real human context for the purposes of demonstrating a grieving person's capacity and willingness to share what for some are unspeakable questions, doubts, and fears.

Presence and Abandonment

Margaret believed in God. All her life she had taken this belief for granted. When she was little, she prayed with her family before meals and before bed. She gave money.

Margaret was almost forty when she overdosed on her medication. She was found just in time. She was taken to the hospital where she remained briefly and then was transferred to a psychiatric unit. This was a traumatic event in a long line of depressive days.

During her time with a counselor, Margaret admitted that she had always struggled to accomplish as much as her siblings. Her mother had died nine years earlier, but Margaret still felt as though she was a disappointment to her mother. She had separated from her husband just before her mother's death, and had known that her mother disapproved of her decision.

Since she had no work experience, and no advanced training or skills, she struggled in low-paying jobs. To add to her burden, she began to feel that her child would be better off with her father. Consequently, she saw her only several times a year. Meanwhile she met a number of men and had numerous brief, but intense, relationships.

Occasionally, Margaret went to church in the town where she had grown up. But, she just didn't feel spiritually nourished the way she had in the past. Motherless, divorced, separated from her daughter, debt mounting, and good jobs few and far between, she began to realize that Jesus was no companion to her. She began to wonder where Jesus was when she needed him. She stopped praying. Going to church was an empty experience that left her frustrated and feeling more alone. It was all her fault. Somehow, she just wasn't one of the people Jesus chose to stick with through the bad times. When the nurse asked her if she had a religious preference, she hotly declared, "Can't you tell? God abandoned me long ago!"

Righteousness and Bad Things Happening

Holly did not believe in God. She often felt left out of group conversations when religious issues were discussed as part of the recovery process. Still, she was a spiritual person and shared that she enjoyed relationships and nature. In former times, beautiful summer days, reading, and art uplifted her spirit. She felt good about herself and her world on these occasions. She could remember feeling righteous, not in the religious sense, but in the sense of feeling that all was right and good in her life. She was confident about the path she had chosen. Life changes brought her to group therapy to explore these changes, her experience of loss, and the overwhelming grief that she could not work through on her own.

Today, Holly was particularly pleasant and active in the therapy session. She supported others and smiled when differences of opinion arose. Everyone in the group suffered from depression. Everyone was grieving significant and often traumatic losses. Everyone was at different stages in the process, and by and large, were able to be supportive of one another. About halfway through the hour, Holly smiled at a group member who had finally accepted that he had a major mental illness. With a calm voice she slowly declared, "You may have a physical illness, but I brought this depression on myself. I made it happen. I was stubborn and mean. Everything that has happened to me has happened because I was bad."

Group members had heard this line of thinking before and weren't about to let Holly escape their gentle, but clear, confrontation. Because she was not a Christian, they tried to express their concerns without using religious language. They told Holly that clinical depression did not happen to her because she was bad, or because she was good. Rather, it was a physiological fact of life that might happen to anyone. Then they suggested that it might be a good idea for her to stop beating herself up. Holly would have none of this. She declared that, "Even in the world of nature, and the best of humanistic endeavors, everyone knows that what happened to me didn't come from nowhere. It had to have been my fault."

Tests and Challenges

Bill lost custody of his children. He had gotten drunk and threatened his whole family. Now he was hospitalized and had a restraining order against him. He missed his children especially. He wondered if, and when, he would ever get to see them again. Still, he wasn't worried because he knew that God was testing him. Or maybe Satan was testing him. Either way, God was allowing it to happen. It was God's will. He wasn't sick, and he certainly wasn't an alcoholic. No way was he going to take those medications. He just needed to believe in God, and pass this test. After all, look what happened to Job.

Suffering, Creation, and Deliverance

"If God loves us so much, why does he let us suffer?" Robert asked the question every session. These days he didn't wait for an answer. "How can they say God loves us? It's just not true. If God really cared, there wouldn't be so much suffering in the world. I don't believe God cares at all. Sure, he made the world, but that was the end of it. Now we're on our own. Nothing, and no one, is going to save us now, so why bother? Look at my dad. He was a good man. He loved his family, worked hard, believed in God, and read the scriptures. Look where it got him. I prayed for him daily, but my prayers sure weren't answered. He died at the age of fifty-four anyway. Did he die peacefully? No way. He suffered horribly. Day and night he was in pain. No matter how much medication they gave him, the pain just kept right on hurting. So I look at it this way: God never had any plan to help us. All that stuff about answering prayers is just hogwash. We're on our own. Jesus may have wept, but that was then, and this is now."

Capacity of God/Higher Power and Use of Miracles

Samuel was the third person in the spirituality and recovery group to wonder why God was so stingy with miracles. "If God is so powerful, why do horrible things happen? Just look at the news. Just look at all the sick, starving, and homeless people. Just look at the abuse and violence. Why weren't there more miracles?" In fact, Samuel prayed for a miracle daily. But none seemed to come his way, from his point of view. He wanted to continue to believe in God, and in miracles, but sometimes, he got so angry thinking about it that he wanted to stop praying all together.

Times When It May Be Too Much to Bear

Tina sat down in the chair. Tears came to her eyes, as she told how much she missed her children and how her husband was going to divorce her. Tears flowed, as she said that her family thought she was no good. Now, she had all these medical problems and wasn't able to work. Quietly, she asked, "Do you think it's true that God never gives us more than we can bear? I believe that. However, this is beginning to be too much."

Commandment to Forgive

Patricia knew that she was supposed to forgive her father, but she just couldn't do it. She still hated him for what he had done to her as a child. Her life was a mess. Now that he was dying, she felt she should let him die in peace. Instead, she imagined dancing on his grave. She felt really guilty for that. Still, she just couldn't forgive him.

Guilt

Marie felt guilty. She had left her young child and escaped to freedom. She believed in Christ and was born again. She talked proudly of her freedom, but still, she felt guilty. She just couldn't get over her nightmares. She vividly remembered the Christians in her homeland who were beheaded. She did not want that to happen to her. She couldn't help but wonder what God thought of her decision.

Spirituality versus Science

George had been hospitalized for a very long time. Most of the time he refused to take medication, or follow other treatment recommendations. When forced to receive treatment, he felt spiritually bereft. He could no longer remember and cite scripture. He could no longer remember the words to hymns that he had known since his youth. During a spirituality and recovery group, he expressed his concern that he still felt called to be an evangelist. He felt profound remorse. He had been harsh in his younger days, when he was the leader of a church. He was proud of how the church membership had grown during his leadership, but he couldn't get past his grief for having developed an illness that made him rigid and angry most of the time. He knew he had hurt people. Still, he felt called to bring people to Christ. Once again, he said that he should not talk about Christ, or the Word, if he wanted to ever leave the hospital. Today, he didn't care. He wouldn't abandon his faith. He knew of people who had been martyred as missionaries. He was willing to die for his faith. He felt at peace with his decision today. Still, he grieved for the ways he had hurt people in the past.

Peter, on the other hand, no longer believed in Christ, or in any religion. He now realized how mentally ill he was, and that he needed to take medications or the psychotic symptoms would reappear. He would put his faith in science. After all, look at what science had done for him. He would never be completely independent again, but his life was still good. He truly grieved what he had done, and felt he had paid the price. He felt lonely at times; that was to be expected. He still attended the chapel services, but he no longer believed in God. Still, he felt good when he was in worship, and sometimes he wished he could still believe in those things.

SPIRITUALLY BASED DYSFUNCTIONAL GRIEF

Examples of Dysfunctional Responses with Spiritual Foundations

Tables 4.1.and 4.2 provide examples of spiritually based dysfunctional grief. In both tables, examples of problems are given based on the locus of impairment, Intimate Spirituality or In-reach, or Transcendent/Transpersonal Spirituality or Outreach.

INDIVIDUALS PARTICULARLY AT RISK FOR SPIRITUALLY BASED COMPLICATIONS

Spiritual beliefs, practices, and life experiences, can place a person at risk for complicated and/or dysfunctional grief. Some spiritual issues are more apt to create complications than others. In all cases, the beliefs, practices, and experiences are based on anecdotal information gained in clinical and pastoral practice. These issues are not intended to be indicators of total functioning, or dysfunction, but pertain to factors that may be present in the spiritual dimension. Thus, they need to be addressed directly, and as part of the complexity of total human functioning during grief.

Belief-Centered Risks

Some people are at risk for complications and dysfunctional grief due to their beliefs. In some cases, the content of a belief can be too rigid or distorted. For others, the belief system is not well thought out, consciously explored, and not shared. Then, there are those times when an individual's beliefs are in flux. Thus, the individual may experience less conviction. He or she may have a deficit in general knowledge and reflective capacity, concerning the specifics of a new system. In some cases, the new belief system is not chosen, and the only current belief is that the old one is inadequate. Furthermore, how one expands on beliefs and processes new information, with additional faith and insight, is crucial for processing loss.

TABLE 4.1. Transcendent/Transpersonal Spirituality or Outreach, Locus of Impairment

Problems	Mild Impairment	Moderate	Severe
Higher spirit/power/ God/God- desses transpersonal goodness	Lack of connec- tion	Denial of relation- ship and influ- ence	Declaration of self as higher power, above others, and/or destructive violence and actions
Spirit of creation	Lack of aware- ness of forces of life, creation, and interdependence	Disregard for im- pact on parts and totality of creation	Destructive acts toward people and other parts of creation such as property
Cultural spirit	Isolation from time, history, and culture	Omission of ritu- als that would normally occur because of defensive responses such as denial and fear of losing control emotionally	Degradation and lack of respect of cultural connec- tions
Communal spirit	Minimization of communal needs Problems asking for help	Failure to take into consideration the needs of oth- ers and the higher good	Prohibition and prevention of healthy responses whether by self or others within one's community Shame
Individual spirit	Mild depression and anxiety Doubts and fears interfere with pre- ferred responses Helplessness	Feelings of guilt and/or worthless- ness	Clinical depres- sion and/or anxiety Sense of impend- ing doom Hopelessness

Individuals Who Have a Negative Worldview

A negative worldview is indicative of unresolved spiritual grief. This negative worldview is usually developed as a result of multiple losses. Great intensity of negativity causes a greater risk for impaired response. A negative worldview can be as mild as a cynical stance, or as severe as paranoia.

Individuals Whose Espoused Spirituality Does Not Include Transcendent or Transpersonal Spirituality

A belief in the interconnectedness of all creation is essential to healthy grieving. Those who do not translate this connectedness to beliefs about relationships, beyond what can be evidenced concretely, tend to have complications during the depression stage of grief. It is essential to sense something greater than self at a time when the self is experienced as vulnerable. As one woman said, "I hand things over to God so that I do not become overwhelmed in anger or anxiety."

TABLE 4.2. Intimate Spirituality or In-Reach, Locus of Impairment

Problem	Mild Impairment	Moderate	Severe
Being and believing	Not attending to daily needs hopelessness	Wish to die Denial of value of self	Suicidal attempts Existential despair
Creating and growing	No energy for change Not seeking help Apathy	Sabotaging attempts to help self and or to let others help	Refusal to change and to learn and to focus on future
Acting and generating	Blaming	Refusal to do what needs to be done	Noncompliance with significant health and safety of self and others Rage directed inward or outward
Witnessing and lighting	Disrespect for others Turning away from own beliefs and principles	Repetition of distorted stories to self and others Stuck in misery Self-centered	Self-flagellation Aggression to self and others Creating havoc and destruction

Individuals Who Have Fixed Thoughts, Beliefs, and Behaviors Within a Personally Codified Belief System

Although it is good to have beliefs, and to act on those beliefs, the more rigid and idiosyncratic the belief system is, the more possible it is to experience isolation, or problems adapting in a world changed by loss. Sometimes a fixed codified belief system brings comfort. However, sometimes a belief system becomes so unique that an individual experiences isolation and frustration in attempts to apply that system to daily living. So, although a certain control and safety is realized in keeping established beliefs, the cost in terms of other relationships can be great. Plus, fixed thoughts, beliefs, and behaviors seldom provide an exhaustive map for new problems and new situations. Thus, the risk is for isolation, repetition of unproductive responses, and problems with accepting beliefs that contribute to an open future.

Individuals in Transition, with Shifting Beliefs

It is possible that beliefs are somewhat in transition throughout life. However, significant shifts in beliefs bring about changes that can result in loss and grief, even when the change is desired. However, large transitions in beliefs can be more challenging when they coincide with significant periods of loss.

This vulnerability was part of Don's experience. He had been raised a Christian and found solace in his faith for many years. However, the time came when he could not believe that God existed, nor did he believe any of the teachings that he had leaned on for so many years.

Consequently, he began to read about other religions. He began to explore what he called "scientific thinking." He was good-natured about this and did not get into conflict with others. He seemed to be happy in this new focus and found some long-sought confidence in his own growth and increased wellness.

One day, however, Don came to spirituality and recovery group and sat silently. He was experiencing a bit of a setback, evidenced by difficulty in concentrating. He also feared that other symptoms were beginning to reoccur. He was worried. Two activities he had found helpful were to focus on a hobby, and to recite Christian scriptures. Both of these comforted him. Sheepishly, and somewhat sadly, he admitted that he was grateful to have remembered certain passages that he could use at this time.

Individuals Who Have to Integrate Traumatic Events into Naïve or Innocent Belief Patterns

Perhaps the spirit is the most traumatized during horrendous events that violate mind and body because trauma is so overwhelming. To accept the reality of trauma, one must accept the vulnerability of life, and the badness, or evil, present within creation. Thus, trauma itself is a spiritually based complicating factor in recovery. Those who have had multiple traumatic experiences are greatly at risk. In addition, a person who is relatively naive, and unexposed to horrendous events, is also at risk for complicated grieving. The leap from naivety to worldly wisdom is a significant leap for which one has no previous inner experience or corresponding spiritual response system.

Individuals Whose Beliefs Include a Closed System of Simple Causality

The postmodern world is complex in many ways. It takes an adaptable mind, body, and spirit just to understand what is happening. Those who think they know how God or a Higher Power acts, tend to believe that they understand the larger picture of divine causality and purposes. Of course this is impossible. When challenged, even the most convinced person knows that total understanding is not part of the human condition. However, when faced with significant losses, people experience new situations that may or may not fit neatly into the closed system to which they currently subscribe. Often this is experienced as an additional loss, and denial regarding this secondary experience begins to take hold. Sometimes the conclusions are comforting and beneficial and sometimes they are challenging and bring about disastrous responses.

Individuals Without a Sense of Individual Responsibility, Autonomy of Choice, and a Version of Free Will

On the one hand, it is helpful to believe in fixed principles that can be remembered and relied upon during calm and stormy times. However, those who feel that everything is controlled by a transcendent or transpersonal power are at risk for either anxiety or depression. The sense that events happen to us, and that we are helpless to change events, complicates the sense of meaning one gains from the grief process. This approach also tends to limit one's initiative to make a decision, to move forward, and to make necessary changes.

Practice-Centered Risks

Spiritual practices can also increase risk for complicated and dysfunctional grief. Although many of us are aware of the consequences of severely pathological practices, grief can be complicated by some of the less severe effects of spiritually based thoughts, beliefs, and behaviors. As usual, there is a tendency to minimize certain practices, or to not follow through with adequate treatment for identified problems.

Individuals Without Spiritual Traditions

In my own practice, I've noticed that more and more people come to work, or to therapy, without spiritual traditions. This appears to put these people at risk for complicated grieving that can begin as early as the feeling stage, and most certainly affects their capacity and selection of resources. In addition, without belief in a Higher Power and a strong sense of morals and values, combined with alienation from friends and family, the grief work becomes lengthier, as this part of spiritual development catches up to other mind and body functions.

Individuals Who Function in Pejorative or Judgmental Systems About Certain Losses or Grief Patterns

A judgmental stance or worldview tends to complicate grief in a number of ways. It often impairs grief when judgment, particularly pejorative judgment, is applied too quickly, and functions as a denial mechanism that limits the construction of reality, the range of feelings, and even the ability to experience genuine sorrow. Sometimes, behaviors that follow judgmental stances can be supported within one's faith group, culture, or community. At other times, the same judgmental stance can put one at odds with others. Furthermore, when a judgmental stance is taken literally, not only are grief patterns upset, but resulting behaviors can lead to negative consequences that set secondary losses in motion, which may actually have an even greater impact in the long run.

Individuals Who Do Not Have Automatic Spiritual Practices and Preferences

The function of automatic spiritual practices and preferences is to provide a quick response to meet a specific need. These practices become ritualized, and in so doing, make coping easier. Therapy helps people not only repair past problems, but also prepares people for, and even prevents, future derailment of natural processes.

Individuals Who Have Become Alienated from Transcendent and Transpersonal Forces and Systems

It is common to confront, challenge, or question transcendent and transpersonal forces and systems. Yet, alienation from these forces and systems is, in and of itself, an indicator of complicated grief that has become dysfunctional. During these times, a person is either stuck in denial or feeling stages of grief, and thoughts and feelings need to be explored. During particularly dysfunctional times, contracts need to be made for safety. It is also helpful to limit behavior while reframing actions that might be impulsive and regretted at a later time. A positive reframe for dysfunctional attitude might include suggesting that the person is a caring person, the person is passionate, or the person probably was doing the best he or she could do. However, the behavior must stop and the thoughts and feelings must be expressed in other ways. One cannot do whatever one feels like doing even if one doesn't believe in transcendent forces, systems, or ethical and moral codes.

Individuals Who Do Not Practice Discernment Regarding Key Spiritual Issues: Guilt, Shame, and Forgiveness

The spiritual practice of discernment is crucial to recovery from significant loss. In this context, discernment is the process of attending to all of the elements of intimate and transcendent/transpersonal spirituality. All information (subjective, objective, or functions of spirit) is the subject of investigation for the purpose of making choices with as high a degree of congruency as possible. Problems with discernment are likely to occur during the depression stage of grief, when insufficient tools exist for sorting and sifting through loss. Problems with discernment are similar to problems with gaining insight and may involve thoughts or cognition. When severe, problems interpreting bodily functions may arise. When spiritual discernment is inadequate, serious problems may develop, resulting in a full-blown disorder.

Individuals Who Distort Sacred Writings As a Defense,
Rather Than Use Them As a Tool or Resource

Everyone distorts incoming data about self and relationship. This happens because all data are subjective, relative, and based on each person's needs. But, some distortions place a person at greater risk than others. In the spiritual dimension, distortions tend to include the following:

- Omission of the larger context in a sacred writing
- Fixation on one tenet or section
- Failure to understand the subtleties
- Concretization of writings that were not intended to be used for the purpose to which they are applied

The distortion of sacred writings usually serves the function of stabilizing a denial system. This effort serves as an indicator of that person's vulnerability. When the distortion helps with the grief process and causes no harm, it is considered benign and not confronted. When the distortion is dangerous to self or others, crisis management systems need to be activated.

Eye for an Eye or Vengeance Response

It is usually a positive sign when a person admits, in the therapeutic and pastoral setting, that he or she really wants vengeance. What is dangerous is covert behavior that must be scrutinized as "eye-for-an-eye" thinking. The subtler the person is about his or her agenda, the greater the possibility for at-risk behavior. On the other hand, violent fantasies do not necessarily lead to violent behaviors. However, it is crucial to consider all thoughts and expressions of eye-for-eye thinking as having the potential for increased risk for dysfunctional grief.

Individuals Who Do Not Normally Practice Altruism

Altruism is an inner spiritual stance of caring for all that exists. Practically speaking, one cares for that which is "other." At its interior base, spiritual altruism protects and develops relationship with spirit, body, and mind. Altruism turned inward promotes care of self, actions that benefit of self, and growth of self-spirit connection. Nonpractice of altruism, in regard to intimate spirituality, can be considered a practice that is either negligent or harmful to self. Non-practice of altruism, within the relational strata of transcendent and transpersonal spirituality, puts an individual at risk for harming others. The degree of impairment, in either case, must be assessed during times of significant loss.

Experience-Centered Risks

All experience is registered within mind, body, and spirit. Each aspect of an experience is stored in a different area with a corresponding coding for access and retrieval of information. Spiritually coded information is gleaned from each experience for the intention of providing meaning, purpose, and connection. The meaning and purpose of each connection that spirit makes may be similar to conclusions of the mind and the body, or it may be different. Hence, body and mind may know one thing, and the spirit knows another. The degree of incongruence, and the importance of the experience, may lead the person to experience greater or less safety.

Individuals with a History of Conflicted Responses to Authority Systems or Rituals

Conflicted responses to events that seem to be autonomous to a person's wishes are a natural part of loss and grief. These conflicted responses may remain until a new stability is gained. The risk of highly conflicted responses surrounding the loss, and how the loss is handled, usually comes from an impaired ability to act, or act appropriately.

Individuals Who Have Unresolved Spiritual Issues
from Past Grief Responses

Unresolved spiritual issues that are part of a past grief may negatively affect present grief. Hence, there may be no time for rejoicing
and recovery. With no rest between losses, one loss can seem like part
of a string of losses. When this happens, the meaning of the present
loss may become distorted. Individuals may develop a sense of negative fate, the feeling that negative forces are at work, or a negative
self-image. These responses are attempts to find the reasons for these
losses. Unfinished spiritual issues also affect the quality of meaning
making that occurs during less stressful periods. Lack of initiative,
autonomy, accomplishment, and general sabotage of best intentions
may result from fragmentation of spirit.

Individuals with History of Complicated or Dysfunctional Grief
Responses Inclusive of Spiritual Impairment

A history of complicated or dysfunctional grief affecting the spiritual area may increase the risk for similar impairment in the future.
Although direct causality cannot be established, many people survive
complicated and dysfunctional grief with strength and a sense of
transformation. When grief has not led to increased insight (knowledge, revision, or strengthening of beliefs), a certain vulnerability to
regression to earlier responses can exist.

Individuals Who Have Been Forbidden to Grieve
Because It Goes Against the Acceptance of God's Will

This spiritual stance serves as a barrier to grief even though it is
disguised in benevolent clothing. Time and again, a Christian who
has prematurely shut down the natural process of grief has done so in
this manner. This response should be respected. At the same time, it
must be considered a defensive mechanism when other evidence indicates that the person has not finished the stages of grief. This is particularly so when one has not truly begun the reorganization stage.
Because this response is intended to prevent the flow to thoughts
and feelings, it causes risk for complications early in the denial stage.
The person then tries to skip thoughts, feelings, the sorrow and sadness, and reorganization processes. When Sherri's mother died she

shed no tears. She accepted the loss of her mother as being part of God's will. There was no need to grieve. She offered this conclusion while in a context that appeared to contradict the possibility that such a miraculous acceptance was coming from true spirit.

In the first place, Sherri was hospitalized soon after her mother's death. In the second place, her father had instructed the family not to grieve. Third, Sherri considered grief to be against God's will. So she said that she had no feelings of missing her mother, for she was in heaven. Sherri was surprised and disconcerted to learn that considerable evidence in Christian and Jewish scripture demonstrated that grief was a common response. Even Jesus wept! Although she wanted to block this information, she listened respectfully to others in the group. She did not change her heart or mind and remained hospitalized, frozen within her spirit.

Individuals Who Have Tried Everything

On one particular day, all three people in loss and recovery group were very depressed. They discussed similar feelings of being in a deep, dark pit. One person felt that there was no need trying to get out of the pit, for each try backfired and even made things worse.

The second person felt that there was no way out of the pit. She said that she was in no condition to talk about it, for that was of no help. She wanted a drink.

The third person, Rodney, had been angry for weeks and was now being discharged. He said it made no difference where he was, for things would be no different.

After a long period of quiet, Rodney asked a direct question: "Do you believe a person knows himself better than anyone else?" The leader agreed with the premise, but added that sometimes we don't know ourselves very well and others have knowledge and insight that we are lacking.

The other two women accepted this observation. But Rodney was headed in the direction he wanted to go. He wanted to confirm his line of thinking. No one had fixed his multiple health problems. Furthermore, since he had been to numerous professionals, he didn't think anyone could.

Deep inside, Rodney still wanted help. His was a spiritual despair that complicated all his efforts to seek and receive help. The risk for people like Rodney is that they feel they have tried everything to no avail. So they make a faulty leap of reasoning to conclude that there is no help. This stance impairs the intimate and transcendent spirit-functions of promoting positive action. Thus, power is transferred to the impaired, distressed function of resistance.

*Individuals Whose Severity of Impairment Is Great
and Located in Several Dimensions*

The referral was for the chaplain to speak with Stacia, who was isolating herself. The mental health treatment team felt she needed more socialization. Stacia was not willing to relate to others because she felt they did not share her beliefs. She was not willing to take much-needed medication.

Stacia spoke with the chaplain briefly, and with great anxiety. In the middle of the brief conversation, her anxiety rose even higher and she blurted out rather loudly, "I cannot talk to you." When asked if this kind of yelling came upon her very often she said, "yes." Then, she calmly stated that she thought God did not want her to talk with people who were not from her church. She said that God was healing her.

Although numerous religious groups feel that it is best to relate to people who are of a similar faith tradition, this factor alone is not a complication. Impairment happens when beliefs actually keep someone from healing by limiting the resources available. In this case, Stacia's faith proved to be tenuous and built on extreme fear and anxiety. Plus her processing of faith and trust in God's healing was limited by drug usage and a growing mental disorder. One of the greatest challenges in situations like this is how to get the whole person working in an integrated fashion. The initial intervention in this case was one of respect and support. Her yelling outburst was only gently addressed and would be followed up on later.

STAGES OF SPIRITUAL GRIEF

In Chapter 1, the six stages of grief were discussed. From that point on, we have seen how grief can become complicated and dysfunctional. We addressed the issues of how complications manifest themselves within certain stages. The following text discusses a model for the spiritual stages of grief. Here we reaffirm that successfully completing the spiritual work in each stage contributes to overall recovery from loss and provides a spiritual model for grief that complements the one provided in Chapter 1. The terminology has been kept generic so that it can be useful to those whose spirituality is expressed religiously or nonreligiously (see also McCall, 1999, p. 157, adapted).

Stage 1: Awe (Shock)

Just as shock signals the presence of loss, so, too, does awe signal the introduction of something new. The purpose of awe is neither negative nor positive, but fact. Awe is experienced as spirit coming upon something that is significant in one's life. Problems registering the significance of a loss constitute a complication in the grief process.

Stage 2: Disbelief (Denial)

Spiritual denial might be likened to the initial process that Moses encountered upon climbing the mountain in the wilderness. Significant losses feel overwhelming and events appear larger than life. They require exertion and energy. Sometimes these events may feel not so much like mountain climbing to face the creator, but more like standing on dry ground that has become quicksand. Thus, even in the presence of something huge we find ourselves saying, "This can't be happening."

Because loss always challenges, and often transcends our expectations, significant loss always throws us into ambivalence. We don't know how to receive the news. We don't know if we should, or will, receive this terrible thing that life offers. Denial and spiritual disbelief gives us room to breathe before we decide.

The spiritual significance of doubt, or disbelief, is to provide protection in case the loss should prove to be too great a challenge to spirit. Disbelief cloaks our fear that we will be unable to protect our established connections with spirit. Disbelief places us upon shifting spiritual sand. Disbelief makes us think that our minds are temporarily in control. Disbelief makes us believe that we can change destiny and that miracles will happen. We prefer to disbelieve the facts of a significant loss rather than wander in a wilderness of confusing thoughts and even more confusing feelings. We think that our disbelief causes us to stand firm. Eventually, disbelief proves counterproductive and we must climb our grief mountains and sink into our spiritual despair. But in the beginning, disbelief helps us feel spiritually safe.

Stage 3: Lamentation (Feelings)

Who has not lamented? Who has not railed when cosmic happenings seem to be personally directed? Who has not lamented the change of seasons, the course of time, the shifting winds, and spiritual happenings that are out of our control? Lamentation is a particular gift that raises mere feelings to importance that transcends self and otherwise seemingly puny human endeavors. To feel is human. To lament is to dialogue with the stars, the universe, and the divine.

Spiritual disbelief, even in the case of moderate questioning, usually leads to feelings about the vulnerability we experience when we are reminded of life's limitations and of our inability to exert control of much of our circumstances. The period of lamentation is our experience of wailing in the midst of eternal power, knowing that we are at the same time subject to all the laws of spirit and creation. However, continued lamentation without cessation leaves a person spiritually raw and wounded. One runs the risk of living a life filled with lament. Spiritual dysfunction at this stage would consist of being left in the depths of Sheol or on the cross without corresponding resurrection. Productive lamentation leads to an experience like that of the psalmist who always followed lamentation with restored belief.

During the period of lamentation, spirit is an active presence. However, sometimes spirit is blocked. Sometimes lament turns to dysfunctional action and impaired relationships. Sometimes lament becomes so overwhelming that nonspiritual resources are called upon to fill the place of faith, trust, and hope. Sometimes drugs, alcohol, and impulsive behavior gain a foothold and distract people from the spiritual grief task of seeking a restoration of their place in creation.

Stage 4: Despair of the Spirit or Dark Night of the Soul (Depression Stage, Part 1)

During the depression stage of grief the spirit knows genuine despair. This provides the spiritual counterpoint, so crucial to reconciliation or recovery. Existential despair is a time of confusion, unknowing, and struggle, to be and let be. It is a strange spiritual fact that surrendering to helplessness is essential to restoration of hope. Some people never leave this period of despair and run the risk of living a life of sorrow that feels like being shackled, or confined, with a shrinking of spirit. Normally, during the process of despair, spirit is companion and comforter. Once a person has moved through despair he or she often knows true grace. If impaired, the action of spirit to companion and comfort is blocked.

Stage 4: Discernment (Depression Stage, Part 2)

The period of discernment marks a time to move from being in sorrow to being in relationship. During this time spiritual connections and spiritually supported relationships are tried, practiced, kept, or discarded. As the loss is processed, so, too, are considerations of the importance of the disconnection and the value of reconnection. During this time, spirit is counselor and guide. Spiritual repairs may be considered. Sins and omissions are owned for what they are. Self-review consists of preparing to take responsibility where appropriate.

When discernment is bypassed, spiritual growth may not occur even when reorganization is undertaken. A certain spiritual shallowness may grow instead. False discernment also leads to impaired responses, just as false guilt and phony forgiveness leave one empty and alone. Choices that don't involve discernment may fizzle from lack of spiritual energy and direction.

Stage 4: Moment of Conversion or Calling (Depression Stage, Part 3)

When the time comes to make a decision to move on, spirit is experienced as the return of creative power and light. The spiritual clarity of such a moment often comes as a surprise or epiphany. For productive discernment leads to empowered understanding and choice in future endeavors. At this point, grief begins to see possible resolution and to know true hope.

Impairment at this stage severely restricts authentic and integrated functioning, and fulfillment as person. Further complications arise when a person feels dragged into his or her future rather than moving into it. Failure to make choices at this point often causes a person to feel especially vulnerable, resentful, and at risk for regression into doubt, lamentation, and existential despair.

Stage 5: Renewal of Beliefs and Practices (Reorganization)

During the spiritual time of renewal, the stance of spirit is that of teacher in relation to disciple. Internal permission is given to learn, grow, and reflect on the journey through grief. This period is usually experienced as a time of openness to new possibilities. At such times, a person has insight into the journey. As with the women on the Emmaus road (Luke 24: 13-35), clarity of experience and continuity of self and relationships begin to return. This is their spiritual experience of renewal following their grief over the loss of Jesus after his crucifixion and burial. "They said to each other, "Did not our hearts burn within us while he talked to us on the road . . ." (Luke 24: 32).

During the renewal process, the person is able to rejoice at having come through the previous stages of grief. There is a realistic appraisal of the importance of what has happened. There may be a treasuring of life that has been lived and the life that one has. Wisdom is often stored so that it can be of use in the future. When the grieving heart "burns with joy" it is because the upside down world of grief has been worthwhile and makes its own kind of sense. Pieces have been put together, not as they were, but as they are.

Stage 6: Healing Connections (Recovery)

One is spiritually recovered when one experiences spiritual well-being. There is enough wellness to celebrate and enough energy to live and do the tasks of daily living. What was a daily burden is a burden no longer. Memories are treasured or taken as is. The promised land of recovery is not the end, but another beginning.

SUMMARY

The spiritual side of loss, grief, and recovery, involves its own pain and challenges. When met with the assistance of true intimate spirit, and true transcendent and transpersonal resources, the process becomes a valued gift, even when it is not chosen. Loss happens, but grief comes to people for the sole purpose of healing. In this sense, grief is one of the many bearers of spirit. Thus, grief is, at its core, a spiritual experience.

Chapter 5

How Perceptions, Thoughts, and Beliefs Influence Care

We use the expression "creating a space for others" to mean that the counselor is ready to be hospitable to the person . . .

Kornfeld, 2000, p. 49

Recovering from complicated grief can be a challenging and painful process. To assist in this recovery task, helpers and care providers need to help the grieving person process and mange his or her perceptions, thoughts, feelings, and beliefs. Once this process is successful, the person can begin to make adaptive and meaningful changes.

During this time of intense internal processing, the grieving person becomes narrowly focused on self. Often perceptions, thoughts, feelings, and beliefs are in flux, turbulent, and, at times, rigid. Thus, the person tends to not be as open minded as she or he might otherwise be. Helpers, and care providers, who understand this necessary time of complete subjectivity, tend to accept that this is a normal aspect of recovery. So they support the process, while still paying attention to the effects on activities of daily living, and the productivity of the processing task.

SUBJECTIVITY, VULNERABILITY, AND PROFESSIONAL BIAS

However, the intense subjectivity of the grief process makes grief work anything but simple. In fact, the process of helping may add to the complexity of grief and increase the risk for complications. While people in need are always somewhat vulnerable to the personality and skills of the person from whom they seek help, certain needs tend to place an individual in a more vulnerable position than others.

The vulnerability of a person, in the midst of profoundly painful grieving, derives from the fact that he or she must delve deeper and deeper into self in order to fully explore the meaning of loss. In the process of painful self-exploration, the helpfulness and stability of all relationships may come into question. Nuances that might have been taken for granted are minutely examined. Trust that might have come naturally now may be measured in a miserly way, for purposes of self-protection. Feelings that might have come and gone in a some-what balanced way may be intensified and displaced on those who are trying to be helpful. In many cases, a dependency on the helper develops. In situations of increased vulnerability and dependency, the perceptions, thoughts, and beliefs of the helper become an even more important factor in promoting healthy grief responses.

Yet, the helper is also an individual with his or her own internally derived perceptions, thoughts, feelings, and beliefs. All of these in-ternal processes and conclusions make up their personal bias or sub-jectivity. The inescapable reality of personal bias makes the learning of grief theory and technique insufficient for completion of the task of training a person to provide services that promote normal grieving, and aid in the resolution of complicated and dysfunctional grief.

All of this being said, it isn't easy to separate one's thoughts, feel-ings, and perceptions, from those of another person, or from the tasks essential to helping. Self-monitoring and growth in this area is a never-ending process required of those who help and seek to do no harm. For, at the same time that one is using oneself to align, under-stand, and empathize with an individual, one is conscious of a man-date to maintain a certain distance and objectivity. This involves get-ting oneself out of the way, while remaining present and available, a paradox integral to all care-promoting endeavors.

RECOGNIZING THE RELATIONAL FEEDBACK LOOP

Perceptions, thoughts, and beliefs form a personal resource that informs current action and is brought forward into new situations. This resource is stored as personal bias. It is a crucial adaptive re-source that promotes quick response, particularly in time of stress.

During difficult times, one's bias is somewhat like a deep well that provides life-giving water upon request. During safe times, an individual might go to that resource and reflect upon its contents (its accuracy, usefulness, and appropriateness). This process of reflection contributes to growth, personal satisfaction, and increased reservoirs of creative spirit.

In helping relationships, each individual draws on this personal bias as resource during a time of identified need—which is usually a time of duress, rather than a time of safety and calm reflection. When these two biases meet, a feedback loop is automatically formed. This basic "helper-grieving person in need of care" dyad, in the form of a relational feedback loop, is represented in Figure 5.1.

In the best of all situations, the newly formed feedback loop promotes a healthy care process that leads to recovery. When this is not the case, the feedback loop is distorted. The resistance of the grieving person to present personal bias, can distort the loop and disrupt the fundamental task of recovering from grief. This is to be expected, and is a basic, natural response during certain stages within the grief process.

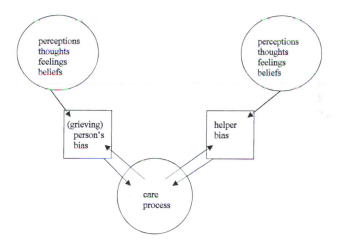

FIGURE 5.1. Relational Feedback Loop

The personal bias of the helper, however, can also distort the relational feedback loop due to inadequate knowledge, self-reflection, or examination, thus contaminating the relational feedback loop. Contamination can lead to narrowness and rigidity on the helper's part. In extreme cases, forcing personal bias on a grieving person can lead to neglect and abuse. Distortion and contamination of the caregiving relational feedback loop is a complicating factor that can lead to dysfunctional responses by all persons in the loop. This contaminated and dysfunctional relational feedback loop developed in Dave's experience with Sean.

Dave, a pastor, never saw his father cry. As a boy, if he started to cry he was told to be a big boy. Big boys didn't cry. When Grandpa Warren died no one cried.

One day Sean sat in Dave's office saying that he had not cried over the death of his father. Dave heard what Sean said, but paid no attention to it. After all, Dave did not think that crying was important, or necessary. So Dave went on with the conversation that was supposed to be focused on Sean's work; besides other things were on the agenda.

Three weeks later, Dave got a call from Sean's wife saying that Sean had been crying uncontrollably and had driven off the road. He was currently hospitalized and facing a drunk-driving charge. Dave thought that all this must have come from something that had happened since they last talked.

COMMON MYTHS AND MISPERCEPTIONS CONCERNING GRIEF AND LOSS

Common perceptions, thoughts, feelings, and beliefs tend to arise during times of grief. As personal bias, these can be particularly challenging and impede healthy grieving. As an aid to recognizing these typical components of bias, a descriptive list is provided in the pages that follow. However, the biases listed are not exhaustive. Those provided are meant to jog the reader's thinking about personal subjectivity and bias.

Examples of the grieving person's bias, and those of the helper, are included even though the primary focus in this chapter is on the helper's bias as tool for promoting recovery. Other chapters focus primarily on the individual's responses. Fundamentally, however, the feedback loop is essentially a relational loop in which both parties contribute bias. Thus both parties' biases are included,

The Grieving Person's Perceptions and Beliefs That Can Contribute to Complications

"That's Done Now"

Carl's grandmother died several months ago. Even though he was hospitalized after a significant suicidal attempt following this recent loss, he declared that he was no longer grieving the death of his grandmother. "That's done now. I really didn't have much grief. After all I wasn't really that close to her."

"I Should Be Over It by Now"

Warren lost his mother a couple of years ago. Since then, he had started using drugs and had been placed on medication for severe depression. During his first group therapy session, he wanted to know how long grief should take. Several sessions later, he continued to believe that he would never recover. He felt he should be over it by now. He believed that continued grief was a sign that recovery would never come to him.

Shelly had a similar reaction. It had been almost two years since her mother had passed away and she remained both angry and depressed. She didn't know why she couldn't just shake if off and get on with her life. She believed it just wasn't normal to grieve this long.

"I Haven't Cried"

Otis had been grieving for several years. He missed his siblings who had died of illness and from an accident. He thought about them daily. He was often angry, confused, and distracted. He stopped going to work, and he slept later and later in the mornings. He was often irritable and increasingly read the Bible. However, when questioned, Otis stuck to his belief that he had not grieved his siblings' deaths. After all, he hadn't cried.

"I'd Rather Not Talk About It"

Paul talked comfortably about most things, expressing his thoughts and feelings. He was willing to examine problems and to consider changing his life in numerous ways. He was bright, affable, and eager to learn, when he was not severely depressed, or when he was asked about his relationship with his ex-wife who had just divorced him. On that subject he declared that talking did no good.

"I Still Get Angry"

Cynthia was sure a mistake had been made when her therapist referred her for loss and recovery. She was adamant that she no longer had a grief issue concerning her son's death. She had done all she was supposed to do. She made the preparations. The service was lovely. She gave most of her son's possessions to friends. She went on with her life. Now, ten years later, a therapist suggested that she had a lot of unresolved anger. Sure, thinking about her son's death still made her angry, but she wasn't grieving. Anyone would be angry! Besides, most of the time she wasn't thinking about what happened. Look at what she had to deal with at work and at home. Anyone would be angry.

"He's in a Better Place"

Stan really did believe that his dying father was going to heaven and that there was no need for grief. After all, he would see his dad when he died. There would be a reunion with all of his loved ones. He shared this belief with his pastor and with the elders. It helped somewhat, because everyone smiled, and said that he was right, and reminded him how important his faith was at a time like this. Still, even though Stan was sure of his faith, and that he wasn't grieving, he felt lonely and irritable. He began to carry his Bible with him everywhere. He even began to talk to strangers. As time went on, he felt called to bring people to Christ. He grew more and more urgent in this mission. He knew there was no way to affect what was happening to his father, still, he reasoned, it couldn't hurt for him to be a better witness for Christ.

"I Can Do It Myself"

Patrick arrived late without Betty. He had just had another argument with her about the divorce agreement. He didn't want to talk, but he worried that it wouldn't look good in court if he didn't continue coming for counseling, so, he showed up. He handed the therapist a check for the session and headed for the door stating, "I can do it myself."

Helper's Perceptions and Beliefs That Can Contribute to Complicated Grieving

"Enough Is Enough—Get Over It" or *"My Way Is the Right Way"*

Patty was tired of listening to her sister whine. This had gone on for years, and enough was enough. Their mother was dead and Sarah should get over it. After all, she had gone though the same thing, and she had recovered. Today, she would confront Sarah with the facts. Life goes on and so should she!

"It's Been Six Months and She Is Not Over It Yet"

Joyce's boss, Mark, had been patient. When Joyce needed time off for her brother's funeral, he had given it to her. When Joyce broke down, cried, and needed to leave her desk, he said nothing. When she arrived late from lunch with red eyes and sniffles, he tried to be sympathetic. But it had been six months, and this had gone on too long. She should be over it by now!

"That's Just Attention-Seeking Behavior"

Kelly was the subject of the treatment team review. Once again, the psychologist brought up Kelly's tears and distress over her father's death. Her father had suffered a painful death several years ago from cancer. Kelly had been hospitalized at the time and was unable to say good-bye. In fact, she had not even known about his death until a week later, because the family felt she couldn't handle it. The psychologist felt that Kelly's grief was a factor in her present hospitalization and that she needed further grief therapy. Kelly's primary nurse, Colleen, disagreed. Colleen believed that Kelly's tears were just attention-seeking behavior. They shouldn't reinforce such behavior. Manipulation was manipulation.

"There Will Be No Grieving When We Go in There" *or "There Are Rules"*

Bertha was embarrassed by her son's behavior. He had lost his dad and she had lost her husband, but there was no use crying. God had taken Vaughn home. It didn't make sense for any of the children to grieve. So Bertha stood in front of the doors at the funeral home and announced to all the children and grandchildren, "There will be no tears." Scott understood his mother. He was supposed to "buck up" and bear it. Inside he felt lonely, angry, and helpless. This feeling increased as the weeks and months went by, but he said nothing.

"He Must Be OK; He Didn't Say Anything Was Bothering Him"

Harold was not one for conversation. He spoke only when he had something to say, otherwise he remained quiet. Everyone knew he was going through a divorce, but that was the extent of it. However, Dorothy, who had an office next door to Harold, noticed that he stayed in his office more and more. The blinds that once were open were now frequently closed. She began to wonder about Harold, but didn't want to barge in if there was no need. Yet, a nagging worry consumed her, so she mentioned her concern to Harold's immediate supervisor, who was also Harold's friend. Greg listened politely and responded with confidence, "He must be OK. He didn't say anything was bothering him."

"Oh, She Talks About It All the Time"

It's true that Betsy always talked a lot. So no one was surprised when she kept talking about her deceased mother. Her mother always did things a certain way. Her mother liked sewing. Her mother would be in Florida this time of year. She had gotten the butterfly pin that she was wearing from her mother. Betsy would talk about anything. If she talked too much, it was best to just ignore her politely, because she wasn't going to change her ways. There was nothing unusual about that.

"It's Best to Say Nothing"

Kurt had been Arthur's pastor for fifteen years. Arthur had served on several church committees and was always upbeat without being outrageous. However, since he lost his job last March he was either moody or off the wall. Either way, Kurt was uncomfortable. Still, his job was to love and encourage members of the congregation. They should come to him if they needed help. So, Kurt decided that it was best to say nothing. After all, Arthur was probably very sensitive to his situation.

"She'll Get Over It"

Martha's mom was not happy. In fact she had not been happy for some time. She missed her husband. They had been married for forty-five years, and it had been a good marriage. He had died in his sleep several years ago. Martha missed her dad, too, but she didn't let it interfere too much with her life and her immediate family. It hurt to know that her mom was so sad, but there was nothing Martha could do. "She'll get over it," she told her husband.

"He Just Isn't Accepting That His Brother Is Sick"

The treatment team was quite aware that Doug had been depressed and suicidal much of his life. This would probably never change. But it was distressing to talk to Doug's brother who just wouldn't accept that Doug was very sick. This all made sense to the team who had worked with Doug for some time. They were a bit annoyed about the brother's stubbornness and resistance. In fact, they were so annoyed that they were caught off guard when the pastoral counselor suggested that the brother was probably grieving rather than just resisting.

"She Just Needs More Faith"

Marla went to see the deacon of her church. She wasn't comfortable speaking with her pastor, but felt that Frank would be a good listener. She was a faithful person and a good parishioner, but she just wasn't up to Father Anthony's challenging of her faith. When she sat with Frank, she shared her anger with God about the death of her young husband and about being left with three children, debt up to her ears, and no job. Frank was a good listener and assured her that there was nothing to be angry with God about. After all, God had not taken her husband, cancer had. Frank said it was important for her to trust God and to pray all the more for help. If her faith weakened, then things would only get worse.

PROBLEMATIC IMPLICATIONS

Thoughts, beliefs, feelings, and perceptions of the grieving person, and of those who relate to him or her, are powerful forces for healing and recovery. Myths, beliefs, and misperceptions, however, can become obstacles to healing and recovery. Unfortunately, many myths and misperceptions about grief are so subtle that they tend to catch people by surprise. Many unhelpful responses are so ingrained that they meet with denial, rationalization, or any available mechanism that serves to help maintain the bias. This is done to avoid change. Because changing certain beliefs and misperceptions can contribute to an additional sense of loss. Hence, there may be an unwillingness to change one's thinking in spite of its theoretical and practical insufficiency.

Problematic Implication 1:
Grief Work Is Not Essential

The myths, beliefs, and misperceptions cited previously seriously undermine the importance of grief work. In this case, the common mechanism for undermining grief work is accomplished through denial and minimization. Subtleties of denial and minimization are found in assumptions about what the process entails—including timing of the process, techniques, its resolution, and purpose. Further obstacles are created through lack of identification of grief, lack of intervention, and inattention to treatment needs.

Problematic Implication 2:
Grief Should Be Simple

The myth that grief is simple impedes the normative process of grieving and undermines the uniqueness of each person's experience. At times, such thinking is evidence of lack of empathy for self or others. At other times, a simplistic view is fostered due to feelings of helplessness that may be brought on by inexperience and the lack of advanced skills. This belief also becomes a rationalization and a cover for focusing on other things that may genuinely be pressing and of importance.

Problematic Implication 3:
Extended Grief Is Evidence of Immaturity or Pathology

Limitations on the process, timing, and resolution of grief may be due to inaccurate assumptions and can lead to further complications and a failure to provide appropriate help. Implications that certain types of processes are not "manly," not mature, or are pathological can result from faulty reasoning—as evidenced in earlier examples. Often, these limitations are due to underlying frustration, anger, fear, denial, and minimization of the grief process and its possible complications. At times, the grieving person and his or her helper are unaware of the depths of feelings that erroneously lead them to place limitations on grief.

Problematic Implication 4:
Grief Is a Way of Feeling Sorry for Oneself
or Getting Attention

This belief is really a subcategory of the previous section. It tends to be a favored variation that can seem condescending or pathologizing what may not be pathological. This belief may be favored because we live in a culture that has always favored rugged individualism and happy endings, whereas the process and individual resolution of grief can be unsettling.

Attempts to stop grief are a normal part of the process of grieving that the individual has to experience. However, when care providers attempt to manage another's grief by suggesting that the grief is not authentic, they are often saying more about themselves and their own needs than the needs of the person. Responses that indicate that grief is self-centered and selfish miss the point. Grief is not so much feeling sorry for oneself as it is experiencing sorrow. During a period of mourning, many people need attention and benefit from companionship.

Problematic Implication 5:
Grief Implies Weakness of Character, Spirit, and Faith

The conclusion that grief represents a spiritual deficit can be most problematic especially when the grieving process is really normal. This approach can be a disguised attempt to limit the exploration of beliefs and understandings that are not always simple or upbeat. Whereas some issues of may evidence immaturity or pathology others are incorrectly perceived as inherent weaknesses in personality and development. When force is at work, people may be judging rather than listening and helping. Weakness of character, spirit, and faith should be explored. But, exploration must not be contaminated by preconceived helper biases. Nor should any of us suggest that we have absolute truth concerning strength of character, the work of individual and transcendent spirit, what faith should be, and how it functions in the life of each person.

RECOGNIZING CRITICAL CARE POINTS

Since grieving is an automatic process set in motion after a loss, it can be said to have a life of its own. Yet paradoxically, this same automatic and even instinctual process is amenable to skilled intervention. The omission of appropriate interventions can increase the likelihood of complications and dysfunctional responses and decrease the potential for healing and recovery. Therefore, it is better to address grief than to do nothing.

One of the most effective ways to remember to address grief is to identify critical care points surrounding the grieving process. Decisions made at these points can sometimes change the course of grief and make the difference between productive and unproductive grieving. However, when these points are missed, the repair work that follows can become an additional complicating factor within the process. Timing is crucial. Critical care points come and go quickly. Hence, they require early, frequent, and consistent attention and a willingness to challenge personal biases that may interfere with their identification. In all cases, courage must prevail to keep one's heart and mind open to the compassionate and healing task at hand.

Critical care points are often overlooked because they make sense. Thus, it might seem that they are too simple to be lifted up and given such a fancy name. However, many opportunities pass us by because we have become so accustomed to them that we hardly notice when they come and go. To counterbalance experiences, beliefs, and perceptions some ordinary moments must become critical care points. Five of these moments are listed as follows.

Critical Care Point 1: All the time
We must always be aware of whether a person is or is not grieving.
We must decide whether a grief assessment is needed.

Critical Care Point 2: When the question of help arises
We must decide whether a person does or does not need help.
We must decide whether help should involve treatment.
We must make referrals for treatment and help select resources.
We must decide whether to include spiritual care or omit it from referral and treatment options.

Critical Care Point 3: When care plans are being made
We must decide whether to develop a loss, grief, and recovery care plan.

Critical Care Point 4: During the caregiving process
We must decide how to use personal bias material that arises.

Critical Care Point 5: At the end of the helping process
We must decide whether to include follow-up care.

At any one of these points, personal and professional decisions are important. At each point, a decision could be made to stop, avoid, or limit a process. These decisions could be crucial to a grieving person's recovery. All of these care points demand discernment on the part of the care provider. None of the decisions made at these points should be forced on an individual except in cases where safety is at issue, and even then, attempts at collaboration are recommended.

USING PERCEPTIONS AND BELIEFS TO ENHANCE CARE

Perceptions are a gift that provide a way to sense our internal and external world. Without this ability to perceive life we would not be able to function, and quality of life would be severely compromised.

However, our perceptions are not necessarily objective. Still, they tend to make sense to us. How we interpret and adapt our perceptions to represent our experiences, and values, speaks of how we use all raw data for the understanding of experience.

For example, Helen Keller was born blind and deaf. Several perceptions had to come together sequentially for her to learn to connect words with experience. First, her teacher Anne Sullivan took Helen to a pump in the yard and poured water over her outstretched hand. Simultaneously, she traced the signing letters for water in Helen's other palm. It was then that Helen make the connection that what she was feeling in both hands went together and formed the experience, and the naming of that experience, as water. Used wisely, our perceptions provide the rest of us the opportunity to help others understand their experiences also.

Perceptions can enhance care and promote recovery by using them thus:

- Make careful observations
- Build relationships
- Further integration and treatment
- Promote professional and healthy behaviors

Use of Perceptions to Make Careful Observations

Noting Obvious, Overt Behavior After a Loss

On one occasion, a nurse was able to save an individual's life by noticing that the person's gait was different, and that his limbs were unusually clammy, even though other vital signs were normal. Plus, a therapist remembered that the individual was often depressed after an encounter with family members. By putting the two observations together, both professionals were able to identify risky behavior that the individual often engaged in after feelings of grief resulting from an interaction with family members. Once this connection was made, care providers changed their beliefs—that there seemed to be no triggers prior to dysfunctional responses. Although grief was not the only factor causing dysfunctional behavior, it was a significant factor that made some responses potentially lethal.

All loss brings change. Significant loss can mean significant change and lengthy grief responses. Purposely paying attention to behavior changes, and noting shock responses, denial, feelings, depression, and even efforts to make changes, can enhance care. The helper's perceptional shift must include a basic understanding that everyone has some kind of loss experience almost daily. This is true even if there are gains. The decision of what constitutes a loss, is a personal one. Since overt changes always mean something, the helper's response must be inquisitive, helping people make links with their thoughts, feelings, and behavior.

Paying Attention to Subtleties

Cindy had been coming to the group for several weeks. She was talkative and demonstrated a somewhat caustic sense of humor. Sometimes, she demonstrated an ability to be quite empathic with other people in the group. Frequently, she would push people away by prefacing her comments with a version of "You wouldn't understand but . . ." This was a subtle pattern that most members appeared to let slide or perhaps didn't notice. One day, she made this statement to the group leader and went on to talk about holding hands with her spouse.

This time, the leader listened to what Cindy had to say and directed her back to the "you wouldn't understand," preface to her narrative. The leader asked what Cindy was thinking when she said this. Cindy glossed over the question and declared that she didn't remember. Meanwhile, she gave a sidewise glance to a peer. The glance had the effect of drawing the peer in and leaving the rest of the group out. Finally, Cindy answered the leader by saying, "You could be empathic, but you wouldn't really know unless you had gone through the same thing." The words were subtle, but when combined with the intimacy of the glance, everyone else in the group realized that one of the complications that had developed from Cindy's years of grief was that she pushed people away before they could get close to her and repeatedly fail to supply her needs.

In order to experience the subtleties of the grief experience, the helper must explore personal losses and processes. In the previous situation, the leader felt pushed back and excluded by Cindy's words and glance. Only by paying attention to that inner response was she able to decide to check out what Cindy was thinking and doing.

This process of constantly observing individual perceptions and responses is tedious, but at the same time, can lead to a breakthrough in a derailed grief process. Cindy applied this approach to her relationship with her spouse and realized for the first time how she tended to verbally and nonverbally push others away and further deprive herself of the intimacy she needed. This approach had been painfully learned in her childhood.

Often, perceiving subtleties of movement, expression, and words can bring one closer to understanding how the individual functions and considerations about what is not functioning well. The same is true of using an intuitive function that formulates hunches about what is going on within a person, a relationship, or environment. Often, the individual accepts his or her current perceptions, thoughts, feelings, and beliefs as truth and has limited access to other possible truths that he or she might hold.

Checking Out Observations

No matter how objectively formulated, our own beliefs and perceptions must be checked out. This involves carrying an internal question mark next to every thought and feeling that occurs—whether internally or interpersonally. The ability to effectively maintain this basic stance is a crucial difference between a novice and a skilled professional. To understand that one knows a lot about grief, and yet in a sense knows almost nothing, puts ordinary individuals in the position of providing extraordinary caring and more meaningful interventions.

Reviewing Inconsistencies and Observing Personal Bias

Current perceptions can enhance care by presenting discontinuity between a helper's thoughts and beliefs, and what is actually being observed. Recognizing this difference opens an opportunity to effectively help the grieving person do likewise. Common inconsistencies are best noted then formulated as questions to ask oneself.

- What am I hearing today that doesn't match up with what I heard yesterday?
- What I see doesn't match what I believe about grief/the person. What do I make of that?

- I am assuming one thing while intuiting that something else is going on. How will I find out more?
- I have so many ambivalent feelings about what is going on with this person. How many of these feelings are mine and how many belong to the grieving person?

In using this approach, personal bias becomes a gauge for testing, rather than a fact for concluding.

Use of Perceptions to Build Relationships

Since most communication is nonverbal, it is possible to conclude that perceptions are the basis for most communication. Sometimes our perceptions aid us in forming closer relationships. Sometimes they impede relationships by keeping us from establishing connections. For professionals, the first task is always one of building and maintaining a specific relationship for the purposes of meeting the service requested or needed.

Aligning Through Identification with the Person

Since grief is a universal response to loss it seems natural to expect that all people can identify with one another on some level. This would be a logical assumption, but perhaps not a realistic one. Unfortunately, many grieving people complain that they do not always feel that others can identify with them, professionals in particular.

For example, a person whose husband died wonders why she didn't get any response from some of their best friends. A person who was sexually assaulted tearfully admits that others seem to be talking behind her back. Yet, they say nothing to her even though she knows that they know what happened. A patient who has been severely traumatized and diagnosed with post-traumatic stress disorder angrily states that the only thing her doctor talks about is that she needs an antidepressant and should enroll in a Dialectical Behavioral Treatment Program so that she can learn to think better and stop being so overcome by her feelings. These may be good treatment ideas but she wishes he would let her talk about her grief.

When we do not let a grieving person get too close to us it is usually because our own issues are getting in the way. When distancing of self becomes a pattern, an open-ended exploration of self is required. Self-reflection and therapy are both helpful. Also, a consultation may be an essential process for the exploration of dynamics that are set in motion within the helping context. The fact is that we usually block, distort, stick to rigid beliefs, thoughts, feelings, and perceptions, because we can identify all too well with what the person is experiencing and we fear where that might lead us. Usually this resistance is due to our own unresolved grief.

Frequently, anticipatory grief focuses on a fear that we might become overwhelmed and not be able to provide professional care. However, being aware of our own grief stories and experiences, and restoring a sense of human connectedness can bring healing to the caregiver and to the person being helped. When we are open to another's grief we are open to their recovery and our own growth.

Being Empathic

People whose grief is profound frequently feel that no other person can truly know what they are going through. Sometimes, this feeling is applied to a corollary belief that attempts at empathy are also inadequate. Just as there is a time and place for every intervention, there are many times when it is helpful to try to walk in another person's moccasins.

Our personal beliefs and perceptions can contribute to our capacity for empathy with a grieving person. Because loss and grief are part of the human condition, this is truly one area where identification with what another is going through can be used effectively. Of course, empathy goes beyond identification and requires the capacity to listen, join, conceptualize, imagine, and feel with another. However, if one has not worked with one's own myths and misperceptions about grieving, one may find it difficult to walk uncritically in another person's moccasins. Yet, in the best of all situations, understanding what has been helpful, and what is not helpful, can be a guide to discovering what would be helpful to others. Even unusually strong reactions to the grieving process of another person can be useful for helping that person observe problem areas.

Treading Lightly and Humbly

One can identify with another person's grief and even empathize with the individual. But, grief is an individual process as well as a relational one. The hard truth is that grief work demands a strict adherence to the principle that primacy of experience belongs to the grieving person. Therefore, respect for the grieving person's autonomy is crucial even when the grieving process appears to have become complicated and responses are dysfunctional.

This respect is essential even when the care provider observes behaviors that are destructive to self or other. Many times these behaviors can be stopped and one can be protected from oneself to a certain degree. However, individuals have the right to their own grief. We can listen, guide, and suggest and express our professional and human opinion. We can even confine people for their own benefit. But, we cannot abuse people by forcing our own thoughts and beliefs on them.

Communicating with Others

Since the grief process responds so readily to listening and sharing, communication is a major vehicle for healing. Bringing communication about grief to a verbal level is essential. Sometimes it is helpful to bring one's beliefs, what one has heard (myths and stories), and one's general perceptions into the conversation for the purpose of helping the grieving person learn, reflect, and share. However, one's personal perceptions must be shared in measured ways and always to the benefit of the other person. These perceptions need to be communicated as personal opinions rather than fact. Just by using this approach, the grieving person is exposed to modeling of communication and given permission to practice verbalizations in a similar vein. Careful attention must be paid to monitoring exactly what is happening within oneself and the therapeutic purpose of any self-disclosure. But sharing does not provide equality between helper and person being helped. The biggest mistake possible is to forget, even momentarily, that our focus must be on encouraging grieving persons to express themselves.

Encouraging Meaning Making

Perceptions are part of the meaning-making process. They provide clues to what is comfortable and what is uncomfortable. They inform us as to attitude and value. They allow us to form hunches about what might be happening inside ourselves and within another person or external context. What we make of what we perceive is our own responsibility. By encouraging the meaning making we encourage others to take in new information, to turn information around, and to question and sort experience. This step is a crucial antecedent to the decision that a grieving person needs to make as to whether to go forward in life in spite of the loss, and in the midst of grief that is unfinished.

Use of Perceptions to Further Integration and Treatment

Thinking Ahead, Noting Problems and Challenges

It is possible to think ahead fairly rationally by using the stages of grief, and by being aware of factors that increase the risk for complications and dysfunction. This objective knowledge is based primarily on theory and professional experience. Sound theory combined with solid practices dictate that patterns are often available to assist in treatment planning. Although grief is not linear, it is possible to predict some challenges, in light of specific information.

Believing that grief can be challenging, and knowing that certain tasks are essential to recovery, can help a care provider glimpse beyond the here and now. It is this practice of strategizing for the future that helps promote safety, and confidence, and engenders hope. Knowing that it is possible to journey through grief can be a motivating and encouraging factor from which others can gain strength and courage.

Documenting Observations, Conversations, and Problems

Making a note of observations, conversations, and problems is both an objective practice as well as a subjective one. The documentation of information gained through use of one's instinctual perceptual process is an important practice that can be undervalued. When common sense is used to make a mental note of what one sees, hears, and intuitively feels, then a simple analysis can provide the additional reflection of "so what." The "so what" reflection leads to the opportunity for something different to happen.

Many people who experience grief are encouraged to keep a journal. This is their form of documentation, usually used for their purposes solely. Paying specific attention to personal losses and identifying grief responses can be a powerful tool for enhancing care of self and others. The professional form of "making a mental note," or journaling, is documentation. Documentation is a more formal way to note observations, conversations, and problems. Ideally, documentation for patient/client/grief care is part and parcel of internal noting of internal responses. Although professionals are not encouraged to keep duplicate professional files of their work with individuals, there certainly is ample space to practice professional/personal journaling, and to keep professional records.

Forming Working Hypotheses

Diagnosis and treatment are built upon hypotheses as to what a person is experiencing. Formulations are made based upon theory, observation, and experience. Our observations and other perceptions become working data for generating professional hunches about an individual's grief process. Coincidentally, the grieving individual has his or her own working hypothesis as to how the process is going. Convincing both parties to accept a hypothesis as personal or professional opinion and not ultimate truth, is very helpful for making room for different happenings. Neither party has the whole objective truth on anything, yet each person's perception and beliefs constitute crucial information that can lead to healing.

Seeking information about childhood and play habits can provide information about a person's capacity to generate working hypotheses about one's world. It can provide important information about how an individual sees oneself in relation to that world. Some people survive by accepting certain events as total reality on all occasions. This is neither right nor wrong. These conclusions may not be distortion but an acceptance of facts that promote survival and should be honored and respected as the reality of that time, for them. But as we grow in our capacity to understand less concrete experiences, our ability to engage in imaginative play helps us realize that seldom are only one or two choices available to us. The same is true of working hypotheses.

In Bonnie's world, there was only one truth, her truth. She was no good. She was an alcoholic and had been so for most of her life. She had no reason to change having lost all that was important to her.

One day, Bonnie's therapist listened to this reasoning while Bonnie was talking with another client. As the conversation continued, it became quite obvious that Bonnie was really just a pragmatic person. Her working hypotheses had helped her survive in an amazing way. But now these same hypotheses were causing her to sink dismally into despair and inertia.

It would not work to be disrespectful about Bonnie's way of surviving insurmountable obstacles. She had done her best and she was alive. Other therapists had tried to confront what they called her "distorted thinking," but they had not walked in her shoes. They had not imagined what life had been like for her. Some had even laughed at her as she stated her beliefs and her theories about herself and her life.

This time, her therapist did not laugh, but asked Bonnie if she played as a child. She was taken by surprise. She was now interested, for the first time in weeks, in what the therapist was thinking. The therapist shared with her the fact that most children are concrete thinkers until about the age of nine. Throughout childhood, play was an important factor in developing imagination, practicing, and providing opportunities for personal meaning making. If she did this kind of imaginative play as a child she could use this skill in approaching her present life. Adults understand that there are usually more than two choices in any given situation. Examples were given.

By the end of the session Bonnie was asked to make a wish. What would she wish for knowing it would come true, just for today? After listening to others make their wishes Bonnie made hers. She had three wonderful wishes. They constituted the first time that she was able to consider the possibility that she might be able to recover. However, even with this progress, Bonnie was encouraged to try out other possibilities.

Use of Perceptions and Beliefs
to Promote Healthy Behaviors

Beliefs can also enhance care. Some helpful beliefs that a caregiver can develop as part of his or her personal bias, and professional presentation of self, include assumptions that:

- Grief is natural: It is part of being human, therefore we all have this in common.
- Grief is relational: It is okay to get help.
- Grief is a sign of caring: It means you or I care.
- It is possible to recover from loss.
- Meaning can be found in the depths of unfathomable grief.

Furthermore, perceptions and beliefs can be useful in the promotion of healthy behaviors for self and others:

- By supporting healthy lifestyles and good self-care
- By modeling healthy grieving
- By providing healthy boundaries
- By lending hope and encouraging renewal
- By retaining humaneness

THE ROLE OF CONSULTATION

Rita, who was Steven's social worker, thought he was a "nice man." Lucille, the pastoral psychotherapist who led the loss and recovery group, found Steven to be somewhat demanding of his wife, with personality traits that made him appear self-centered and extremely needy. Rita shared her empathic position with Lucille and said she agreed with Steven that his wife did not need to be going to school at this time. Lucille was surprised.

From Lucille's point of view, the same information meant that Steven's wife was going to school during the week, coming home to take care of their children, and working on the weekends. She also visited her inpatient husband. Steven wanted her to quit school and be with him.

As the conversation progressed, Rita noted how her viewpoint differed from Lucille's. Consequently, Rita thought more about her response to Steven. In turn, Lucille considered her alignment with the spouse.

It is probably true that neither Steven nor his spouse are completely right. Both were grieving a relationship that was not working well. The brief consultation between the care providers did in fact help both understand how they had absorbed and adopted parallel viewpoints. Rita agreed that Steven needed his wife's attention and that her school wasn't as important. She therefore identified with him. Lucille realized that she had become empathetic with the spouse who was doing everything and still coming to visit her husband. These thoughts, perceptions, and beliefs helped to encourage Steven to explore his internal grief, and work with his spouse regarding their relationship.

Consultation is an essential process in promoting healthy grief processes and use of self. When formal consultation is not available, three standard questions can be used to uncover personal and professional bias.

- What am I paying attention to and am I taking something for granted?
- Am I uncomfortable and what is that discomfort about?
- Am I helping the person and the grief process or am I getting in the way?

Even in cases where the answer to each question is "yes," the response is always unique to the person asking the question and the presentation of the grieving person.

SUMMARY

The purpose of this chapter has been to further the understanding that myths, beliefs, and perceptions influence responses to loss and grief. This is true of the grieving person and of those who strive to be helpful. Although some beliefs and perceptions are helpful, others tend to contribute to further complications. Certain points in the grief process are considered critical care points, as the decisions made at this time tend to affect the outcome of interventions. Personal beliefs and perceptions of the helper can also, paradoxically, complicate grief and have the potential for enhancing care.

Chapter 6

Therapies and Treatment Priorities

There's a story about a woman with a serious case of hives who went to see a specialist for relief. She had suffered much, living for some time in continual pain, because the hives covered most of her body. She needed healing, and hoped that the doctor could prescribe a cure. But his diagnosis surprised her. "There is no physical reason for your hives," he told her, and then paused. "So, it's my conclusion that your skin is crying because you cannot."

Hershey, 2000, p. 95

On a cold and icy day at the beginning of a new year, an admissions team in an acute care psychiatric hospital gathered to do an exit interview with a middle-aged woman. A member of the team began the interview by asking the woman what she had found most helpful during her hospitalization. The woman was doing quite well and spoke openly with affect, "I found everything helpful." A team member went on to encourage the patient to be more specific: "We really want to know what you found most helpful during your hospitalization." The woman thought briefly, and said with conviction, "The loss and recovery group. I have been grieving so many losses for so many years that I couldn't recover from any of them. This group helped me start to recover."

Three years later, another middle-aged woman complained about a change in services in a local health care program. For many years, the community mental health center held services for its clients upon the death of one of its members. However, this time when a member died, clients were informed that services were no longer provided. No explanation was given. There would be bereavement groups, but no services, religious or otherwise. The woman was distraught. She felt that the services had helped her through many losses, and she had difficulty getting the same help in the bereavement groups. "No one will talk to me about this," she sighed.

> *The primary goal of treatment is the movement from complicated/dysfunctional grieving to normal/functional grieving.*

The goal of treatment for complicated and dysfunctional grieving is to help the person return to functional (albeit painful) grieving. In Chapter 2 the grief response service wheel was introduced to demonstrate the continuum of grief from normal through complicated and dysfunctional responses. The wheel also demonstrates the importance of specific treatment interventions as the grief response becomes more complicated. Ideally, the services provided would help the grieving individual return to normal grieving, which then leads to recovery.

> *A primary indicator of recovery is the return to a healthy lifestyle.*

Since recovery is the desired outcome of all grief work, it is crucial to be able to identify what constitutes recovery. Although the task of defining recovery seems challenging, the best definition is the simplest one. The least helpful definition suggests that a stationary state of being exists that does not include the gains and losses of everyday life. Rather, recovery includes the periods of time when one is experiencing everyday losses that may be painful and frustrating but that are not significant enough to interrupt life functioning for more than perhaps a day or two.

For example, a recent trip to have my hair cut confirmed suspicions that my hair was getting thinner, making it difficult to hold a permanent. To make matters worse, the news meant a change in my hairstyle. So, I left the shop sporting a much shorter style that I equate with little old women. The experience was shocking. For a day and a half, I went through all the stages of acute grief. Thus, I experienced a larger loss of well-being, and a continued grief about being middle-aged. These losses raised additional unresolved grief issues. Nevertheless, the change in amount and character of my hair is one of those everyday losses that happened in the midst of a period that, by and large, was marked by life satisfaction or recovery.

The greatest indicator of recovery is the return to a healthy and positive lifestyle. This includes the experience of being connected to others, and of having a strong desire for living, hoping, and dreaming, as well as pleasure and creativity. In some cases, the return to a healthy lifestyle requires movement in a direction in which a person has not been functioning for some time. When this is the case, therapy must continue and reparative work is needed. This type of reparative work focuses on losses that are usually experienced over a lifetime, may be traumatic, and often result in the uncompleted developmental tasks, or in managing problematic personality traits. Losses in these situations tend to be losses of potential to be the person that spirit has intended the person to be.

TYPES OF TREATMENT

Primary treatment for grief recovery is talk therapy. Adjunct therapies are often essential for complicated and dysfunctional grief responses.

The primary treatment in grief recovery is talk therapy. Through communicating one's thoughts and feelings with a compassionate and skilled person, the grieving individual is able to express himself or herself and experience renewed connection. Expression of self does several things. First, it provides catharsis or the discharge of feelings that have been internal and sometimes unaccessible. Second, talking provides the externalization of thoughts and beliefs that can be sifted through and sorted. Finally, talking gives the individual the opportunity to prioritize, plan, and practice thoughts, feelings, and behaviors, thereby making external changes along with internal connections.

Several factors need to be present for therapy to be helpful. First, the person must be allowed to express and experience his or her own reality. This reality must be received empathically and validated as the truth for that person at the time of expression. Validation must verbally and nonverbally complete a communication feedback loop. In addition to this initial and sustaining connection, the therapist, or helper, must convey a sense of confidence in the possibility of recovery and an ability and willingness to be a skilled guide and companion during the process.

This being said, numerous therapies can be applied to the treatment of grief. Some therapies are appropriate for certain grief stages but not for others. Plus, some therapies work better with some complications and dysfunctions and are not as successful in other instances. Typically, therapies are chosen based on the skills and training of the individual therapist or helper. This is often the result of the pragmatics of who is contacted, whose services are reimbursed or privileged by third party insurers, and the preferences of those who refer. However, the skilled professional will take into consideration factors such as the focus or outcome of each specific therapy, the length of treatment desired or available, and of course the proven usefulness of each therapy.

A part of almost all therapies is devoted to helping with the management of grief. In most cases, this is because some loss is involved whenever the services of a professional therapist, pastoral care person, or other helper/care provider are requested. The following treatments are arranged according to type—basic grief, adjunct therapies, longer-term therapies, and multiple therapies. Each type of treatment is then presented according to modality, length of treatment, type of therapy, setting where therapy is conducted, and use of therapy.

All of the following therapies have been used to help individuals through complicated and dysfunctional grief responses. Each one has its strengths and its limitations. To assist in the understanding and selection of therapy, the following format is used as a template.

Treatment modality
- Therapy names
- Focus of this type of therapy

Length of treatment
- Brief, acute—one to three months
- Moderate—three months to one year
- Long-term and/or continuing care—over one year

Types of therapy
- One-on-one
- Group
- Family/couples/partners

Setting
- In community
- Outpatient
- Inpatient

Use
- Normal grief
- Complicated grief
- Dysfunctional grief

Limitations and treatment issues

Two treatment approaches are designed primarily to help individuals recover from grief and loss. The first type of therapy is a version of talk, or narrative, therapy. The focus here is on giving the grieving persons ample opportunity to talk about the loss and their grief. The therapist listens and uses common therapeutic techniques to help individuals explore all aspects of the loss and the manner in which grief is working itself through. In the second type of treatment, psychoeducation, the grieving person is taught that grief is normal and that typical phases, stages, and tasks need to be worked through in order to recover from loss. Knowledge of these stages helps the person feel less isolated, more accepting of self, and aware of barriers to recovery.

LOSS-FOCUSED THERAPIES

Narrative Therapy

Focus. Narrative (talk) therapy focuses on talking about a loss or losses. The narrative addition to talk therapy utilizes the all-important aspect of telling one's grief story. The process is experiential, relational, and provides ample opportunity to practice new versions based on shifting thoughts, feelings, beliefs, and experience. To this end, the therapist notes shifts within the grief story and reflects these observations back to the individual. During the second half of the journey toward recovery, the grieving individual is taught to observe and reflect on his or her own story, and to practice making changes within the therapeutic context. The stages of grief are sometimes used as a resource to assist in the grieving process.

Outcome. By telling and retelling the loss story in the context of another relationship, the experience of loss and grief evolves over time.

Average length of treatment. Brief, moderate, and/or long term

Type of treatment. Group and one-on-one

Setting. Inpatient, outpatient, and in community

Useful for. Normal, complicated, and dysfunctional grief responses

Limitations. Talk therapy may be sufficient in itself. Additional therapies may be needed, particularly when complications and dysfunctional responses are severe. However, story is still the basic foundation for other therapies as well.

Some therapists may choose to limit talking about loss in the free-form fashion important to telling one's story. This can present an issue for those engaged in structured therapy, or those participating in multiple, concurrent therapies. For example, a woman had difficulty talking about her grief. She kept insisting that, "Some people say, 'get over it.' " She realized that this meant, "Don't even talk about it." She said her current therapist preferred her to focus on the here and now. Although this response may block the natural healing process in the long run, it can be addressed in narrative therapy by talking about the priority of treatment scale presented later in this chapter.

Psychoeducational Therapy

Focus. Psychoeducational grief therapy focuses on teaching the stages and processes of grief.

Outcome. The grieving person learns to identify grief responses and where he or she is in the grief process. Furthermore, the person is taught to recognize complications and barriers to recovery and as a result, can learn to seek resources and be an active participant in his or her own therapy and recovery process.

Average length of treatment. Brief

Type of treatment. Group, part of one-on-one focus

Setting. Inpatient, outpatient, in community

Useful for. Normal, complicated, and dysfunctional grief responses

Limitations. People who are not reality oriented, or who have severe personality disorders that are not being managed well may be problematic participants in group therapy. People who are developmentally challenged may need additional one-on-one support or expressive therapies. Some latitude needs to be provided for teaching management of feelings, monitoring depression, and limiting problematic behaviors. Aggressive and very angry people may need to tell their story even in the midst of the educational part of the group. Otherwise they have difficulty attending to information that is being discussed. Ideally, narrative and psychoeducational therapy are used together.

ADJUNCT THERAPIES

Whenever complications arise within the grief experience, more than one treatment is often helpful. Choices of adjunct therapies are based on therapeutic need, the focus of each therapy, and its intended outcome. Individual personalities, preferences, and styles may also be considered. Most therapeutic modalities address loss and grief, but current preferences include behavioral therapies, holistic therapies, expressive therapies, and systemic therapies that focus on working within systems and relationships. Also, medications may need to be used. The grieving person may also have substance use issues that arise during the grieving process or are preexisting factors that inhibit recovery.

Behavioral Therapies

Cognitive Therapy

Focus. Cognitive therapy focuses on the restructuring of thoughts designed to change distortions and eliminate, or neutralize, unhelpful thoughts surrounding loss, grief, and recovery.

Outcome. Changed thoughts change affect. Changed affect changes behavior and experience.

Average length of treatment. Brief

Type of treatment. Group therapy, from time to time, may be part of one-on-one therapy

Setting. Inpatient, outpatient, and in community

Useful for. Normal grief, helpful for complicated grief, essential for dysfunctional grief responses

Limitations. Cognitive therapy does not address meaning and value sufficiently. Confronting denial responses too quickly can cause more resistance. Challenging or limiting affect too quickly can cause feelings to escalate. Distortion that arises from a therapist's point of view may negate a person's reality and the very real impact the past may have on the present. Cognitive therapy needs to be used with narrative (talk) therapy, or taught as a separate tool.

Counterfactual Therapy

Focus. Counterfactual therapy focuses on confronting the reality of questionable facts by providing consistent alternative information. This can be a more challenging version of cognitive therapy in which the therapist knows the truth. All alternatives to the truth are blocked.

Outcome. The person is compelled to face certain objective realities of a loss.

Average length of treatment. Brief, reinforced long term

Type of treatment. One-on-one, occasionally in group therapy

Setting. Inpatient, occasionally outpatient

Useful for. Dysfunctional grief responses and helping those who are severely impaired, as well as people who cannot comprehend a significant loss. Those who remain in denial may benefit from counterfactual therapy.

Limitations. The person needs to be able to withstand reality confrontation. Resiliency needs to be assessed, with an eye to regression or further dysfunctional behavior. Confrontation must be made in the context of a perceived caring relationship.

Problem-Solving Therapy

Focus. Problem-solving therapy focuses on resolving day-to-day difficulties and solving specific immediate problems.

Outcome. Problem solving is meant to limit dysfunctional behaviors and manage complicating factors that are barriers to current functioning.

Average length of treatment. Brief

Type of treatment. Group therapy, may be part of one-on-one therapy

Setting. Inpatient, outpatient, and in community

Useful for. Working with normal grief responses. May be helpful for complicated responses. Is often essential for dysfunctional grief responses.

Limitations. Problem solving does not lead to integration. It does not promote a larger picture of life, or of the meaning and significance of loss and recovery. It does temporarily address impaired behaviors, including inappropriate expression of feelings. Learning a process for problem solving can become a helpful tool for addressing problems during the reorganization stage of recovery.

Stress Reduction Therapy

Focus. Stress reduction therapy focuses on learning coping skills through use of stress reduction techniques.

Outcome. Stress reduction can lead to decreased vulnerability to internal, relational, and environmental stressors.

Average length of treatment. Brief

Type of treatment. Group and/or part of one-on-one therapy, self-help, health and wellness programs

Setting. Inpatient, outpatient, and in community

Useful for. Normal grief, helpful for complicated, and essential for dysfunctional grief

Limitations. Stress therapy does not work directly on grief, however, it can temporarily reduce symptoms so that a person can use other therapies and resources for grief work.

Holistic or Mind/Body/Spirit Therapies

Pastoral/Spiritual Care Counseling

Focus. Pastoral psychotherapy and spiritual care counseling, promote the integration of grief recovery process through an exploration of questions of meaning, purpose, and connection.

Outcome. Increased inner connectedness and relational stability

Average length of treatment. Brief, moderate

Type of treatment. Spirituality and recovery group and/or one-on-one therapy

Setting. Inpatient, outpatient, and in community

Useful for. Normal grief, essential for complicated grief

Limitations. A pastor, or spiritual care provider, who is not a clinically licensed therapist can provide pastoral counseling. When this is the case, careful attention must be given to the skills and training of such a care provider and to the possible need for additional therapies. On the other hand, "pastoral counselor" is also a term used to describe individuals who are certified therapists comparable to any mental health counselor (see following section on pastoral psycho-therapies). Spiritual guidance is not a substitute for therapy for persons whose grief response is complicated and/or dysfunctional.

Existential Therapy

Focus. Existential therapies focus on the integration of the grief recovery process within the larger context of life and human existence. Existential therapies have been particularly helpful for survivors of very traumatic events in which human value and existence is threatened.

Outcome. Increased sense of self, as part of human condition, with emphasis on connectedness, higher human principles, and altruism

Average length of treatment. Brief

Type of treatment. Group and/or one-on-one

Setting. Inpatient, outpatient, in community

Useful for. Normal and complicated grief

Limitations. The grieving individual who responds best to this type of treatment tends to be well educated and functioning well prior to the loss. Some aspects of this treatment are useful for people recovering from traumatic, horrendous life circumstances, and for generational challenges. At some point, the choice of personal response must be based on a transcendent or higher sense of meaning and value. However, this value can be found in the smallness of ordinary of life that can also seem miraculous. This valuing of small and greater aspects of life makes this approach helpful to all people.

Alternative Spiritual Care Therapies: Meditation, Labyrinths, Spiritual Direction, Religious Counseling

Focus. These therapies focus on exploration of spiritual meaning through religious and spiritual resources, practices, and rituals.

Outcome. The person experiences connection with transcendent and higher powers that serve as companions, guides, and saviors/helpers, through difficult times resulting in a decrease in isolation and feelings of aloneness in grief.

Average length of treatment. Brief, moderate, long term

Type of treatment. Group and/or one-on-one

Setting. Inpatient, outpatient, in community

Useful for. Normal grief, helpful for complicated and dysfunctional grief

Limitations. May change affect, and isolation, and provide containment in painful times. Individuals need additional therapies to provide clinical assessment and help for complicated and dysfunctional responses. Helpers providing these resources may have limited mental health understanding and may be cooperative, or pejorative, of other essential therapies.

Expressive Therapies

Art Therapy, Body Movement and Dance Therapy, Journaling and Poetry

Focus. Expressive therapies focus on the expression of grief through a variety of senses and mediums other than verbal.

Outcome. The individual learns creative ways to express grief and receive catharsis.

Average length of treatment. Brief

Type of treatment. Group and/or one-on-one

Setting. Inpatient, outpatient, and in community

Useful for. Normal, complicated and dysfunctional grief responses. Expressive therapies are often essential for those whose verbal responses are compromised, whose dysfunctional behaviors escalate in conversational therapies, and who cannot process grief through other direct verbal means due to stage of grief and/or intensity of trauma.

Limitations. Whenever possible, interpretation and feedback are useful tools that promote the cognitive/affective understanding of loss and processing grief. In nonverbal cases, the therapist needs to have a basis for understanding the grief expression of each individual and channeling it through the medium provided. In some cases, other behavioral therapies need to be provided.

System Therapies

Focus. System therapies focus on the understanding of familial and communal systems and their effects on personal grief.

Outcome. The increased ability to work within a system to get one's needs met in constructive ways.

Average length of treatment. Brief

Type of treatment. Group, one-on-one, family, and couples/partners

Setting. Inpatient, outpatient, in community

Useful for. Normal grief, helpful for complicated and dysfunctional grief responses

Limitations. Since systems therapy focuses on relational patterns, the individual must have the capacity to differentiate self from others. Psychoeducation about stages of grief needs to be incorporated. The application of systems work to the grief process must remain clear. Further therapy may be needed.

Medication Therapy

Focus. Medications are used to stabilize dysfunctional responses, whether thoughts, feelings, or behaviors.

Outcome. Medications provide the individual with sufficient physiological help to process grief.

Average length of treatment. Brief, moderate, long term

Type of treatment. One-on-one

Setting. Inpatient, outpatient, in community

Useful for. Complicated and dysfunctional grief responses. Medications may be temporarily used for normal grief responses when the loss is traumatic/particularly challenging.

Limitations. A medical doctor, or qualified practitioner, is needed for this therapy. A psychiatrist is an important resource for people with major dysfunctional responses. Medications need to be monitored. Medication is not sufficient to resolve grief, nor does it work on the grief itself, however, it provides a more stable foundation so that grief can be experienced and explored.

Substance Abuse Therapy

Change Therapy

Focus. Change therapies focus on understanding the stages of change and their application to recovering from substance abuse.

Outcome. Increased awareness and practice of recovery from substance abuse

Average length of treatment. Thirty to sixty days, throughout life-time

Type of treatment. Group

Setting. Inpatient, outpatient, in community

Useful for. Normal, complicated, and dysfunctional grief responses

Limitations. Substance abuse therapy is not sufficient for grief work. However, this therapy may be a necessary first step in cases where the substance severely inhibits processing and insight. Treatment for substance abuse alone will tend to be regressive if grief work is not also undertaken.

LONGER-TERM GRIEF THERAPIES

Individuals who experience moderate to severely complicated and dysfunctional grieving often need to commit themselves to longer-term therapies that focus on insight and integration of the past, developmental tasks, and growth of personality. Since this is often repair work, the process can be intense. The person must be somewhat stabile, or be able to use behavioral techniques to maintain appropriate functioning. People who benefit from long-term grief therapy tend to have concurrent illnesses and traumatic, multiple losses.

Psychodynamic Therapies

Focus. Psychodynamic therapies focus on insight, understanding of patterns and internal processes, integration of functioning, and the ability to understand and care for self.

Outcome. Improved self and relationships

Average length of treatment. Moderate, long term

Type of treatment. One-on-one, occasionally group

Setting. Group, one-on-one, in community

Useful for. Normal and complicated grief

Limitations. Person must be able to tolerate the tensions of self-discovery and the limits set on internal, immediate, gratification of needs. Requires investment of time and money. Those who undertake psychodynamic therapy must have the desire to change and grow.

Developmental Therapies

Focus. Developmental therapies focus on insight and growth, based on integration and of self through the various developmental stages of life.

Outcome. Developmental stage repair (including completions of earlier tasks) and advancement in level of age-appropriate maturity

Average length of treatment. Moderate, long term

Type of treatment. One-on-one, occasionally group

Setting. Inpatient, outpatient, and in community

Useful for. Normal, complicated grief

Limitations. This therapy is best undertaken during the sorting process of the depression stage, and when working on reorganization stage tasks.

Holistic or Mind/Body/Spirit Longer-Term Therapies

Pastoral Psychotherapy

Focus. Holistic therapy focuses on integration of self through insight, change, self-development, and repair, with additional focus on integration of renewed sense of meaning, purpose, and connection, at all levels of being.

Outcome. Ability to be authentic self in relationship to others, environment, and transcendent/higher reality

Average length of treatment. Moderate, long term

Type of treatment. Group and/or one-on-one

Setting. Inpatient, outpatient, and in community

Useful for. Normal grief, essential for complicated grief

Limitations. The therapist must be a licensed or certified therapist with skills in clinical as well as spiritual repair/therapy. The grieving person must be open to holistic healing and transformation.

MULTIPLE THERAPIES

Multiple, Concurrent, and Sequential Therapies

Focus. Selection of appropriate therapies based on multiple needs

Outcome. Integrated treatment program

Type of treatment. One-on-one, group

Setting. Inpatient, outpatient, in community

Useful for. Complicated and dysfunctional grief responses for major mental illnesses—such as clinical anxiety, depression, and post-traumatic stress disorder

Limitations. Multiple, concurrent, and sequential therapies require close management and consultative processes.

ESTABLISHING TREATMENT PRIORITIES

Treatment priorities are the same for grief and loss therapy as for any other treatment regimen. Although grief can seem like a circular process, it happens within the individual mind, body, and spirit as well as within relationships and multiple environments. This complex context for grief can be a factor in promoting rapidly changing affect and functioning. Therefore, careful attention must be paid to safety, the individual's capacity for self-care, and the care of dependent others, as well as to the more verbal and affective internal processing of grief.

Treatment Priority Scale

- Safety
- Functioning
- Grief processing

Safety

A person's safety is assessed based on desire, access, or plan to engage in harm of self or others. Safety can be an issue even though some self-harming behaviors may be subtler than others. For example, a diabetic whose blood glucose is very high may cope with a loss by eating carbohydrate-laden food that drives blood sugar higher. Individuals who become so angry with life and losses, and engage in road rage that places themselves or others at risk, present both a safety and functioning problem.

Functioning

Adequate daily functioning is also taken into consideration. Assessment of daily functioning notes degree of impairment, availability, and use of resources. Safety and functioning go hand in hand. The degree of dysfunction and the area of impairment are examined when deciding whether thoughts, feelings, beliefs, and behaviors also raise questions of safety.

Grief Processing

Grief processing focuses on identifying losses, understanding these losses, and gaining insight into their effect on oneself and one's life. The individual learns about complications and dysfunctional behaviors, then seeks to resolve and change those things that it is possible to change, and let go of those that cannot be changed. At times, a person learns how to carry grief and not have it continue to interfere in negative ways. This process is actively engaged in when a person is safe, and functioning is not a significant issue. In some cases, resources can be used to ensure greater safety and limit regression while processing grief. Despite treatment priorities, grief processing must always consider functioning and safety.

A HOLISTIC TREATMENT PROCESS

All therapy is about recovery. Some therapies are about repair and development and other therapies move beyond recovery, repair, and development to focus on growth and transformation. All of the therapies mentioned in this chapter help the grieving person do at least one or more of the tasks of repair, development, recovery, growth, and transformation.

However, some treatment processes focus on a narrower part of this process than others. Thus, it is important to continue to stress that no one therapy is sufficient to resolve complicated and dysfunctional grief. Therefore, a grieving person must have access to several professional resources and receive treatment from an individual proficient in several types of therapy.

Unfortunately, terms such as recovery, repair, development, growth, and even transformation, do not tend to motivate most grieving individuals, or therapists, even though most people like to have things neatly organized and broken down into discrete tasks. However, there is a way to use clinical language and still reach a desired outcome. To this end, it is possible, and even worthwhile, to reframe the task in more meaningful ways that will generate energy and promote hope while accurately describing this very human endeavor.

In the following section, the treatment for grief is described according to a holistic understanding of the primary task and objective of grief work. The phrases used to describe this task and objective are integrative phrases that can be empowering, educational, transforming, and avoid some of the resistance sometimes encountered in more traditional models. In this case, the holistic treatment process does not change the need for, or use of, the more traditional stage process, but rather enhances it according to larger functional treatment perspectives.

- Primary Task: Remembering Well
- Primary Objective: Continuity of Being
- Treatment Steps: Remembering Well and Reconstruction of Continuity of Being

Remembering Well

Many people feel that the purpose of grief is to allow a person to let go and move on after a loss. Therefore, the commonsense admonition is to "forget about it." In response to this admonition, the grieving person often declares, "I can't."

Strangely enough, the grieving person is correct when following this instinct. However, being correct does not take away the pain, nor does it answer the question of what to do with an experience that cannot be forgotten. During normal grief, the conflict resolves itself and time tells how the experience is perceived. During complicated and dysfunctional grief responses, the challenge of whether and how to forget is intensified and often becomes another barrier.

Therefore, this holistic model recognizes that one cannot just forget about important losses, or the attachments that were so important, or the pain of grief. Accepting this truth, another therapeutic approach is offered. This approach focuses on helping the person *remember well* all that there is to remember. This is not a simplification of the task. Rather, it is a respectful, realistic assessment of what needs to happen for recovery to begin.

To complete the task of remembering well, the individual must explore all avenues of memory, experience, thoughts, feelings, and spirit. To these personal experiences, one must add all information that can be provided from as many resources as possible. The journey of comprehensive remembering is an extensive one that is accomplished through commitment to knowledge, growth, and understanding. In many cases, the task of remembering well requires an exhaustive search of present and past, of generations, and of connections with wider contexts and higher processes. The task itself is probably never fully completed. In fact, it is often placed on hold many times until new understanding and experiences develop and information and insights break through. Often changes in life, developmental stages, and anniversaries move the task of remembering to new levels. Affectively, *remembering well* moves from the processes of acute grief through varying degrees of anger, sadness, disappointment, relief, and even exhilaration, as the task takes on new avenues of expression.

Continuity of Being

Remembering well leads to an ever-increasing sense of *continuity of being* which is the objective, or desired outcome, of holistic treatment. It recognizes the essential human status that we are who we are. Thus, all of what we are is both minute and cosmic in context. This gives us ample room to grow, understand, and learn. This gives us room for amazing possibilities. As a result of *remembering well,* during grief, we return to the "us" we know and move toward becoming who we will be in our future. We do this to the degree that we are increasingly aware of the "us" we have been in the past.

In this sense, *remembering well* begins as a task motivated by an experience of profound loss and fragmentation. This loss and fragmentation generates a process, or vehicle, for wholeness and increased wellness. This is so because recovery from grief, when seen as the experience of remembering well, is a helpful way to understand the past, live in the present, and move dynamically into the future. This continuum, or continuity of life, is essential. All of life has history as well as future. Most people instinctively know this fact.

Those who experience connections often want more. They feel nurtured and supported. Their life takes on greater meaning. This is true because connections are crucial to human living. In fact, being connected is the basic state of human stability. Disconnection brings grief; connection brings joy. When connection can no longer be accomplished in former ways, it must be done internally and within the broader text of being more fully human. Thus, memory can be a gift.

Treatment Steps Toward Continuity of Being

Although a specific process for remembering well remains in the developmental stages in this text, some steps appear to be crucial to meeting the overall objective of continuity of being. Experience dictates that these steps are not meant to be strictly sequential, but, rather, represent a template that lends itself to a holistic treatment process. However, the process of remembering well always begins with remembering and all of the other steps become action statements that correspond to essential movement and energy.

Step 1: Remembering

One must remember the thoughts, feelings, and essence of self in relation to the loss. This step always includes the use of narrative to begin to tell the story of loss and grief. Efforts are made to listen to the specific story of what happened, when, and how. One focuses on thoughts, feelings, and beliefs about the loss and the grief process. Many times the story is told as though it was scripted. Other times, one is barely able to tell even a small part of the story and may choose to not speak about it or to talk around it.

Step 2: Containing

The process of containing helps the person find and develop the capacity to remember thoughts, feelings, and the essence of what was, and what is no more. This next step involves listening and perhaps inquiring. It involves encouraging the person to tell his or her story. It also involves assuring the person, verbally and nonverbally, that, whatever the story is, it will be listened to and respected.

The helper or therapist must somehow convey to the person that (no matter how difficult the story is, no matter how unbelievable, no matter what kind of loss) his or her story is important enough to be told. This begins to build a sense of trust and safety that are the containers essential to facing the seemingly unbearable.

There is a sort of rhythm to building a containing context for remembering. Sometimes the therapist asks the person to go as far as possible. At other times, the therapist suggests that the person pause and maybe take a deep breath. At times, the person is encouraged to take time to find the desired words or feelings. Sometimes, the therapist wonders about a deep thought and brings it to the person's attention. At other times, that thought or feeling is not addressed.

Many times, a transitioning or coping technique is taught in the midst of a particularly anxious or depressive moment. The most helpful transitioning technique is to suggest that the person change the subject for a bit or practice thought stopping. The person is assured that these transitions are not meant to suppress thoughts and feelings but simply to hold them until they can be expressed in a safe way. On all occasions, the person is encouraged to decide when to stop, or to continue, thereby enlarging the capacity to contain grief.

Step 3: Deepening the Well of Feeling

The expression of a wider variety of feelings helps the person move deeper and deeper into the complexity of these thoughts and feelings until the solid bedrock of one's humanity is reached. The well of feeling is not deepened by the simple expression of feeling, no matter how strong. Rather, the well of feeling is deepened by gently pushing deeper into feeling, and beneath feeling, until one has reached the depths of one's being.

The beginning feelings of grief are often anger and sorrow. The well of feeling is deepened when nuances of anger are sorted through— annoyance, disappointment, frustration, and so on. The well of feeling is deepened when fear is found hidden under a disappointment that has been hidden under sadness and depression. The well of feeling is deepened according to the number of authentic feelings that are experienced and shared.

Step 4: Enlarging the Space Through Pondering and Wondering

A space for pondering and wondering is created through a two-part process. First, the person experiences the closing in of thoughts and feelings. These thoughts and feelings become so narrow that the person's focus and experience is reduced to the basics of human experience. At times the interior space is so constricted that the person feels selfish but can't do a thing about it. When this happens, the person will often try to enlarge his or her space by pushing against these thoughts and feelings sufficiently to make room for new thoughts and new feelings. This is the second part of the process. The more complicated and dysfunctional the grief, the more challenging it is to find interior room to embrace the magnitude of what has happened, and, therefore, accomplish the task of remembering well. As paradoxical as it may seem, complications often make one feel as though one is what one thinks, feels, and believes. This occurs because of a reactive/protective response to find safety during shifting times.

Interior space can be enlarged, externally, in the beginning of the helping process by encouraging a person to sit, to be, and to share what can be shared. The therapist models the enlarging of space by leaning forward, opening his or her stance, and changing position through a receptive placement of hands, head, or arms. The therapist also enlarges space by teaching, by encouraging conversation in a number of areas, and by switching from direct conversation about loss to other seemingly unrelated areas that may involve learning, beliefs, and other concerns. This must be done tactfully, while piquing the person's interest as to where the therapist is headed.

It is not sufficient to ask open-ended questions of people whose grief is complicated. This procedure can be highly threatening and increases anxiety. A more effective approach is to occasionally wonder or to imagine how the person might feel.

For example, an individual who was recently referred to therapy started to get defensive when asked how she was doing. She became more defensive when asked if she had experienced recent losses, and became clearly agitated when it was suggested that she was referred for therapy because she might have experienced losses. No way was she going to engage anyone in the group. At this point one of the leaders suggested that it must be difficult to come into a group and be asked questions. The dam burst. To this statement, she responded that it certainly was difficult and she thought it was a worthless endeavor (although she actually used stronger words than this). With her therapist she was used to just talking while he listened. This approach was different and she didn't like it.

Genuine affirmation and amazement at a person's struggles, accomplishments, or coping strategies often enlarges one's interior thinking. Often individuals feel they have had little or no choice and can only see their struggles and experience a sinking sensation. Allowing and encouraging expression of feelings about the helping process can enlarge one's space.

Step 5: Making Meaning

Meaning is made as the person builds an understanding of the totality of memory, thoughts, feelings, and relationships that make sense, at least for the time being. This understanding is then stored as a new reality that contributes to movement and development of spirit. The meaning that comes during the early stages of grief is sometimes true (makes sense to the person) but not necessarily true forever. Lasting meaning is essential to stability of self in the world. This is not to say that meaning does not enlarge itself in a revelatory way, but rather that meaning is paradoxically permanent and shifting at the same time. Meaning can only exist as energy and life-giving spirit as a result of soul or spirit-filled introspection, reflection, and as it makes sense in the larger contexts of life.

Step 6: Monitoring Change

It is important to pay attention to what happens when new meaning takes hold and adjustments are made based on current values and beliefs. Loss usually brings undesirable changes. When this happens, change becomes part of the grief experienced and requires its own reflective processes.

Usually initial change due to loss produces anger and protest. At some point in the grieving process, it stops being threatening and an empty lull settles in. Denial decreases. Feelings have been expressed. Information has pretty much all been gathered. The person is confronted with the choice to either complete the grieving process or to stay in sorrow or mourning.

During this lull, the person finds no safety in former feeling, realizing that all has been done that could be done within the protective system set in place to adjust to the loss. Some people say they feel depleted, empty, wrung, comparing this feeling having just competed in an athletic marathon. This time, they know they cannot rail against the loss any longer and need to face change. Although this is part of depression, it is not the early part, but rather the letting go, just before the leap to grasp their future.

Ideally, the grieving person uses the therapist as guide more than companion at this point, so that he or she can practice making choices and living with these choices. When helping a person monitor change, it is helpful to empower the person to try out choices, as long as these choices do not seem to be unsafe or have permanently harming consequences. Thus, the person learns to monitor all choices of thinking, feeling, believing, and acting, in terms of how well these choices are working for him or her.

Step 7: Creative Expression

Creative expression helps a person face the future with increased energy to be and do. Creative expression is an important step in the process of holistic treatment because not all action is of equal importance to spirit. Much of what we do is basic to life. Some of what we do is not truly important, but part of habit, or a reaction to realities that are not authentic to our self. The purpose of reorganization, after a significant loss, is to find new ways to connect to self and others, or at least to experience a rebirth in significance in who we are in the world. Creative expression deals with fostering and practicing all the ways we put meaning into life. Meaning is the inner energy, and creative expression is the light from that energy.

Step 8: Continuity of Being

The experience of continuity of being is the experience of all that was, and is, and makes up who one is today—including those persons, dreams, and even important things that have gone on before. Sometimes, a person who has gone through a difficult experience will say, "I feel like I'm back to my old self." This is not to be taken literally, for the person knows that he or she is not the same as before.

Usually the expression means, "I'm back!" This statement implies that what happened (usually change, loss, grief, healing, recovery, or new directions) made the person feel as though life had taken a detour, or a turn, and was not on track. When the new track is put in place, it is made up of some of the pieces of the past. Thus change and continuity occurs that is comforting and makes sense—continuity of being.

SUMMARY

While the focus of holistic treatment is on the grieving person, the helper, or therapist, not only guides the person through the steps of remembering well, but does so only by going through his or her own parallel steps. It is important in grief work that the helper also do what the grieving person is being asked to do. This makes complicated grief work not appropriate for all clinicians, clergy, or other providers.

The grief journey cannot be just observed, nor can one rely primarily on empathy. In the world of grief, we are all companions on a similar journey. Our stories are our own, but the paths of our journey have been well tread by all of humanity. All the more precious is the sharing of this journey.

The challenge for those engaging in grief work is to truly be there while reserving a part of self and spirit to wander ahead, help to clear the path, to find protection in the forests of fear and pain, while staying just a bit behind to consider how to help the person heal the wounds that have become infected by factors and actions that still leave their sting in heart and soul.

Chapter 7

Positive Strategies
and Helpful Interventions

... the task is not one of installing hope as much as evoking it, calling it forth from the clients' own rich resources. You may lend hope to a client who has little, but it is only a loan. ... In this sense hope is not given as much as found. What we give our clients is, at most, a lens or mirror through which their own vision is clarified.

Yahne and Miller, 2000, p. 229

Charlene came to the group willingly. She participated in the discussion, supporting others as she identified with some of their symptoms and behaviors. Midway through the hour, she reminded the leaders that she had lost her grandparent six months ago, and now, more recently, her mother. She was estranged from her father whom she had never felt close to during her childhood years. She talked of her grandmother. Sadness and laughter combined as she described a loving, and at times totally contradictory, woman who helped her mother raise her. Then she spoke of her father. She told of family secrets, and of information that had been told to her about her father's behavior. She had learned things about her father that she had been far too young to understand, let alone handle emotionally. She wiped tears from her eyes.

She remembered being told about her father's infidelity to her mother when she was twelve. She didn't remember what she had thought or felt. She guessed she was in denial. She could say no more on the subject. A few minutes later, after listening to others talk, she started to tell her story again. "I've always been a bad girl, a problem child." She stated this with conviction. Then she went on to talk about all the trouble she had gotten into as a child. She had done mischievous things that any child might have done. She had been punished by a swat on the seat of her pants, or by having to stand in the corner, or, by missing some special event. "Now my dad won't have anything to do with me. He won't believe I've changed. He won't forgive me."

Charlene continued to have a twelve-year-old view of her separation from her dad. She thought she had done something wrong and that was why he did what he did and left her and her mother. Now, as she neared thirty, she still told the story of her loss and grief from the experiences and conclusions she had drawn as a twelve-year-old all those years ago.

Charlene's story may seem similar to other stories. Yet, her story and her grief are unique to her. She may, or may not, have told this story before. But this time, when Charlene was telling of her losses and her grief, she was doing so with peers who were there to help her. She was also telling her story in the presence of a trained grief therapist. Thus, the story had become larger. Now, the group members were becoming a part of her story; she was in the midst of people who were intently focused on hearing and helping her without being too caught up in her previous experiences.

In this experience, the therapist used a technique for enhancing self-discovery. The purpose of this technique was to trace the beginning of Charlene's grief story. She was asked to remember when she first heard the horrible news about her father's infidelity. At first, Charlene did not understand what was being asked and could not offer the information directly. Rather, she provided what is sometimes called a derivative statement. She gave information that demonstrated the result of the question asked. She started her story again, "I've always been a bad girl . . ."

Unconsciously, she provided the information requested. Through gentle exploration, she was eventually able to hear that she was twelve when she first created the painful grief story that she told that day. The story always began the same way. Thus, the acting title continued to be, "I've always been a bad girl." This title was always followed with the story of her estranged relationship with her father. Because she continued to tell the same story, her grief always seemed to be the grief of a twelve-year-old. With this fixated grief story, it was no wonder that Charlene had the sinking feeling that her grief would never change.

Once the connection made sense to her, she thought about this new piece of her grief puzzle. Then she asked the group, "If I wasn't a bad girl, why did my father leave?" At this point the grief process began to flow once more. From here on, she was free to consider other information and to sort through other experiences that she had access to as an adult. Thus, she began to move into the sorting phase of depression with fresh energy. A very important complication, the memories and conclusions of a twelve-year-old, were now a part of the process but not the whole process.

GENERAL GRIEF RESOLUTION STRATEGIES

The various strategies presented in this chapter will all follow a similar format. A composite vignette will be used to present an important therapeutic issue relating to complicated and dysfunctional grieving. A small part of the process for working with the person will be included in the vignette or discussed afterward. This format will provide an opportunity to look over a helper/therapist's shoulder to hear people tell of their loss, their grief, and of the complications that develop. Sometimes these complications will lead to extremely dysfunctional grief responses.

The examples of interventions used to respond to grief are intended to broaden the therapist or helper's understanding of experiences of grief, and suggest possible ways to engage the grieving individual. In this way, the helper or therapist is able to gain new skills, sharpen a few older ones, and enlarge his or her own story. As with grief therapy, the approach is neither sequential nor linear. Rather, grief therapy is a relational event that moves in somewhat predictable as well as mysterious ways, bringing new life and the possibility for new experiences.

STRATEGIES FOR TELLING THE GRIEF STORY

Grief resolution begins with an experience that is stored in body, brain, heart, spirit, and in affect, as a memory. Memory and story are the same when the story is being formed and told. The experience of loss initiates the beginning formation of a grief story. Whether this story lives, or becomes fixed and rigid, depends on many factors that have been previously noted. In one sense, the task of the helper or therapist is to assist the movement of grief stories by facilitating the process of remembering, and supporting the individual's experience of being an integrated and authentic part of his or her own story.

Initially, the grief story needs to be told thoroughly. This can take a very long time and requires many repetitions, additions, and renditions. The helper's primary task is to strategize the best way to hear, empathize, and respond to the story. This is true no matter how many times the story is presented. The task of the grieving individual is to tell his or her story. In the beginning the story is told with the hope of experiencing relief from painful thoughts and feelings. Later, the story is told to develop insight and find meaning. Then, after some time, the story is told because of its potential to bring change. Finally, the story is told to retain continuity of being throughout life.

Thus, one always begins with the grief story. Initial strategies must focus on facilitating the telling, and nonverbal, expressions of this story. The five following strategies are addressed directly to the person who is helping the grieving person tell his or her story.

Use the Grief Story to Get Close and to Develop a Caring Relationship

Sophia could not talk about her grief, so she kept the time short, never going over fifteen minutes and always watching what others were doing around her. She was on the younger side of midlife and still struggled with an eating disorder. She focused much of her attention on authority issues that she was experiencing with hospital staff. They were holding firm. She was standing in place, also. She was nice about it, but nevertheless, she and the team were at odds. Thus, in the beginning, Sophia's story was very limited. It was, in fact, limited by the events and moods of the day and the moment. This was a grief story that appeared to have no past and no future.

For months, it seemed as though therapy was going nowhere. Some problem solving, stress reduction, and relationship building occurred. The therapist came two times a week for one-on-one therapy and Sophia attended loss and recovery group two times a week.

The rest of her treatment regimen was medical. Her parents visited frequently and she had only good words to say about them.

About six months into treatment, Sophia began to talk about her life prior to hospitalization. She spoke about her education and her work skills and experiences. After a year of therapy, she began to talk about her life when she was no longer working. She spoke of a time confined to her parent's home, and focused on her image, weight, and food. Soon after that, she was telling and retelling her story in a more complete manner.

By the end of one and a half years of intensive therapy, Sophia disclosed something that the therapist could react to in a passionate, and compassionate, way. She spoke of how her parents had watched as she was dying. This part of the story the therapist found horrific and said so. Sophia had not thought of the time and the event in a similar way. She was surprised by the therapist's response.

At this point, the therapist was appropriately fond of Sophia and cared a great deal about her. The therapist was intensely committed to helping Sophia recover and thus had a healthy grief response to Sophia's story. The therapist was shocked, couldn't believe what she was hearing (denial), and became internally angry on Sophia's behalf. This grief response was shared, in a limited way, with Sophia, as a way to help Sophia enlarge her story and model how a story can change with hindsight and insight. This intervention proved to be a turning point.

The therapeutic relationship lasted for two years. During this time, Sophia worked hard and began to create a new story that ended with living, rather than with dying. When this shift occurred, Sophia proceeded to grow up, and no longer needed inpatient treatment.

Positive Strategies

- Encourage the telling of the story.
- Give the person ample time and space to tell his or her story.
- Accept what the person can, or cannot do, at any given moment.
- Allow yourself to be moved by the story. Respectfully add some of that feeling to help the person move the story along.
- Find specific ways to demonstrate engagement in the grief story and care for the person.
- Model healthy grief.

Accept That Telling the Grief Story Is Therapeutic

Norm was a veteran. During the Vietnam War he spent his service time in Germany. After he came home life seemed to go downhill. He had difficulty in his job and with relationships. Occasionally, he needed mental health services. The person screening Norm for post-traumatic stress disorder felt that Norm probably didn't have it. After all, Norm had been nowhere near the battlefield. He probably was just looking for another answer to his health difficulties.

However, Norm was sent to the post-traumatic stress disorder (PTSD) educational program. In the beginning, Norm was cautious. He admitted that he expected the leaders and the group to minimize his military experience. He told some of his story in a cautious manner, checking around the room to see how people responded. His experiences sounded traumatic and people in the group said so. During the second session, he told more of his grief story. By the third session, he seemed to gain energy and insight.

In reviewing the program, he stated that it had been helpful to know the facts, to know that he had PTSD, and to accept that perhaps he had another mental health disorder. He said it was a relief to have people listen. This was the first time he felt that that he could tell his story about the numerous traumas he had experienced throughout his life. He was amazed that everyone listened and seemed to hear him. He felt that the group understood some of what he had gone through, and what a burden these experiences were for him. "Now," he said, "I can finally understand some of the effects of that traumatic time in training in Germany, and how awful it was to come home. Now, I believe I will be able to talk about this more clearly with the people I love."

Telling the grief story is not just a technique to gather information that is then used in a therapeutic manner. The act of telling the story is, in itself, therapeutic. This is the most powerful grief intervention available no matter how normal or complicated the grief process.

Positive Strategies

- Stay in the "here and now" of the story.
- Set aside information provided by others as hearsay until the primary experience of hearing the story has occurred.
- Support the story. It belongs to the person, and is of value.

- Even if the story is not objective truth, it represents the true experience and memory in this moment.

Recognize That the Task Involves Hearing, Listening Well, and Becoming an Advocate

Jordan was young. He had tried every medication he had been told to try. Some of the medications had side effects that he just couldn't bear. Other medications made his symptoms worse. Some medications were tried more than once. Now, his doctor was suggesting that he try something else. His patience was thin and his anger grew: "Just tell me one new medication that I haven't tried." Needless to say, the doctor was discouraged about Jordan's attitude and maintained that medication was appropriate and a better one could be found.

Later, the treatment team discussed Jordan's reluctance to taking further medication. The grief therapist stated her observation also: "He sounds discouraged as well as angry. He must be frightened and probably in his grief doesn't even recognize that what he's really saying is that he feels scared and helpless. Those are hard things for a young man to admit." The therapist had been listening to Jordan and to the treatment team, and they weren't really at odds even though they thought they were. They were both interested in treatment. Neither party had a complete sense of what would work. Both realized that past treatment had not worked as well as hoped.

But this time, listening led to a change in how to interpret the information being gathered. Within the framework of loss and grief, Jordan's response to treatment made sense and needed to be taken seriously as a grief story in its own right. Once this grief story was heard, Jordan was referred to loss and recovery group to address grief issues concerning his illness and the course of treatment undertaken to date.

Positive Strategies

- Listen for what is beneath the words and affect.
- Search for common humanity and lift it up.
- Listen to facilitate the completion of a communication loop and empower the grief story.

See That Words Are Delivered Well, and for a Good Purpose

Dennis suffered from a deepening depression. In addition, he was experiencing relationship difficulties that might lead to separation and divorce. He was scared. However, to his credit, he was motivated to work. He just didn't know what to do, or even how to begin. After a few group therapy sessions, he realized that he had a history of multiple traumatic events and that he met all the criteria for post-traumatic distress disorder. His grief was profound. He was referred to a psychoeducational group about PTSD that he found helpful.

As a result of the sessions, things began to click for Dennis and he felt hope begin to build. However, contact with his spouse left him in panic and emotional pain. He asked for an appointment with the group therapist and talked about his fears tearfully. In the midst of telling his story, he stopped and said, "I guess you don't know what to say."

It so happened that the therapist had indeed been wondering what to say and took her time choosing a response. "I think by now you know that I don't just say things to be positive, or to gloss over what is happening." Dennis responded, "I know you don't, that's why I asked to see you." At this point, he relaxed. The rest of the time was spent discussing what had happened, what might be going on, and how Dennis might manage his energies, and his fears, while retaining hope.

Dennis found this exchange meaningful because the words had a ring of truth that was simply and nondefensively stated. The success of the strategy depended on a relationship that had been established, and on a sense of timing and delivery that was focused and respectful. Sometimes words are true but timing is poor. Sometimes words are spoken when it is a time to be silent. In this case, silence and words both promote recovery.

Positive Strategies

- Ask the person if the story has been told to his or her satisfaction.
- Consider whether the words you have said or omitted are authentic.

- Pay attention to the responses that follow all interventions and adjust your strategy accordingly.
- Think about what needs to happen first. Make sure you are aware of the primary issue.
- Help the person stop and transition if overwhelmed.
- Strive for honesty and integrity as therapist.

Make Sure to Provide Nourishing Words

Words need to be aptly spoken and carry meaning. Such words are nourishing. In the previous example, the most hopeful moment came later in the session. Dennis had begun to worry and wonder if he could complete the program that he was going to undertake. He asked the therapist what she thought. She told him that she believed that he could do the program. She cited specific examples to back up her belief. These examples were observations about his demonstrated capacity and motivation to engage in therapeutic processes and programs.

The therapist suggested resources that would also be nourishing to Dennis in his new program. These resources were cited to form a bridge that Dennis could use during the transition time between one program and another. Some of the resources would help him learn more about male relational issues and masculine development. Another was a good recovery self-help book. A suggested resource to help maintain and develop his spiritual dimension was provided. He responded positively to this and especially identified with the suggestion of maintaining his faith. Both he and his therapist felt that Brian's spiritual life and practices were essential additions to his life and his new treatment plan. After all, with his relationships in stress, his faith in God would be all the more needed.

Positive Strategies

- Try to provide resources that meet the specific needs of the person.
- Consider whether what you have to say is valuable, i.e., helpful.
- Have something to offer.
- Make referrals.
- Remember achievements, no matter how small, and lift these up.

- Recognize and accept your limitations.
- Have cognitive educational resources handy.
- Affirm problem-solving skills.

STRATEGIES FOR DEVELOPING A SENSE OF SELF

The self is always in flux, alive, and in a process of renewal. During grief, the self is thrust into a new experience that is uncomfortable and may challenge some, or all, that the self considers its own. Complicated grief strategies are designed to help the person recognize that he or she may be fragmented, wounded, and even working unproductively (even though the self is continuing to strive to complete its primary functions that would, normally, tend to foster wholeness). One of the therapist's/ helper's primary tasks is to find a way to understand the person, view the person as he or she views himself or herself, and help the person develop in productive and meaningful ways. Strategies, that are useful, empower self to work on its own behalf. To this end, the following strategies are suggested.

Look for Evidence As to How the Self Is Developing

Stephanie could not get over the death of her mother. It had been a long time and she remained in a mildly depressed state. She could work and take care of the family, but she no longer felt joy in doing so. She continued to feel a large hole inside her that couldn't be filled. In the fall, she would think of the holidays, making presents, and large family meals. Much of the season she felt tearful. She was a child without a mother. It wasn't supposed to be this way!

In the winter, she was cold and angry about the snow, and the ice, and being cooped up with the kids on snow days when they couldn't go to school. Her mother had made those days special for her and for her children. Her mother had always brought games and projects, like making cookies, to a dreary winter snowbound day.

In the spring, she missed gardening. Her mother had lived down the street and always planned her garden as well as Stephanie's. When Stephanie's husband suggested they take a cruise, she refused. After all, her last trip had been with her mom to Europe. Just the two of them!

Of course summer was problematic. Most of the season had been spent at her parent's summer home, what with Stephanie not having to work in the summer. Now, she just lay around the house, with the shades drawn, unless the kids got on her case.

This was just a small part of Stephanie's grief story. She brought it to group several times before someone said, out of desperation, "Did your mother go to bed with you too?" The comment felt cruel and Stephanie was hurt to the core. Next week she reported that she couldn't get the comment out of her mind. Once she got over the outrageous insensitivity of the other group member, she was able to think about what the member might have been trying to say. Sheepishly, she looked at the group leader and then at the rest of the group. "Today, I'm not going to talk about my mother. I'm going to talk about me. I don't know me, I guess. At least, I don't know me without my mother."

In a group session, all participants are grievers and all participants are helpers. Often, the leader's role is to help the group do its various roles. Sometimes, this means directing the focus and flow of the group, and sometimes it means getting out of the way and letting events follow their course. Often, there is a need to respect the wisdom of all people in the group, when it comes to grief. After all, members, including the leader, have had losses and grief responses. All members have stories to share about what they have tried, and what has helped or not helped them. Of course, when the leader is also a therapist additional skills lend to the process—such as clinical knowledge, spiritual knowledge, process understanding, and the ability to assess individual strengths and needs. Stephanie needed to grieve the loss of a very dependent, but good, relationship with her mother.

Possible Strategies

- Use the group to seek differing responses. Help people reflect on differing thoughts, feelings, and beliefs.
- If a person is psychotic, or highly emotional, find the threads that point to emotion and support the feeling level. Continue to assess possible behavioral consequences.

- Whenever possible, support attempts to get through situations while recognizing that some of these attempts may not have been the best choices, given hindsight.
- Look for a place to suggest options, choices, or the practicing of new thoughts and behaviors.
- Feel free to participate in brainstorming and hypothesizing. These tools may enlarge a constricted sense of self and context.

Help the Person Recognize and Develop Differences, Preferences, and Clarify Inherent Styles

Denise lost her grandmother whom she loved very much. Denise considered herself blessed. Her grief story began long before her grandmother became ill because her grandmother helped raise her. She loved the memory of the time spent with Nana over the years. She remembered the huge breakfasts that Nana made. She laughed when Nana encouraged her to watch her weight as she loaded the plate with sausage, pancakes, and syrup. She wept when she told of the day that Nana told her that she had cancer and wouldn't live long. They hugged each other and both cried. To the very end, Nana listened to Denise's every interest and every story, adding praise or encouragement. Nana marveled at the few interests they had in common and at how assertive and outgoing her granddaughter was.

The day of the funeral, the whole family gathered back at Nana's house. Denise felt strange and bewildered. Everything was the way it had always been except Nana was no longer there. Denise found herself looking for Nana around every doorway, but to no avail. It had been almost a year and Denise still missed her grandmother intensely. However, she found herself coping and going on with life. She actually was seeking help for herself now. She had been told that she had cancer and she was worried and scared. She found herself thinking of her grandmother and drew comfort from knowing that Nana's spirit was guiding her. Denise knew she had to make her own choices, but she tried to think how supportive Nana would be of any choice she made, no matter what the consequence. She knew, at least intellectually, that her present task was to focus on herself. It was hard to do.

Whenever one is separated from a loved one, a profound change occurs that must be addressed for healing and recovery to occur. Individuals who are too independent, and have difficulties with attachment, struggle to understand the connection that has remained unconscious and therefore inaccessible. Individuals whose lives are so interconnected that there is little individuation, and much dependency or enmeshment, also struggle to find who they are without the other person. Either way, loss means an adjustment in the understanding of self. If a new sense of self is not beginning to form by the time the individual reaches the depressive, or sorting stage, then sorrow and sorting may remain incomplete, or less productive. Until the self reasserts, at the time of the "decision to go on," then reorganization is stalled and sorrow is likely to deepen. Disease and dysfunction are possible complications.

A sense of self is renewed, developed, and repaired through the grief process.

After the initial shock, denial, and early anger phases, it is always helpful to encourage the grieving individual to focus on inner thoughts, feelings, and beliefs. Further interventions that encourage identifications of differences in preferences and style, also encourage development of self. This would include asking the grieving person to talk about the loss, and about others, from a more objective standpoint. For example, after a grief story is completed, Stephanie might be asked, "What do you make of the role your mother played in your life?" Dennis might be asked, "How did the medications affect who you want to be as an individual?" Denise might be asked, "Two years from now, what would you like to be able to say about the choices you need to make now?"

Possible Strategies

- Teach the person to identify differences, preferences, and style.
- Begin by subtly noting where these aspects can be referred to within the person's grief story. However, don't do this during the first telling of the story, nor in the midst of extremely painful or charged moments.
- Be sure to occasionally wonder about a person's assessment of another person's thoughts, feelings, and behavior. Ask the person to clarify knowledge she or he is asserting about the other person. Accept answers without further investigation until the relationship is sufficient to contain room for wondering about grief facts and conclusions.

Increase Complexity Through the Multiplication of Specifics Unless Otherwise Indicated by Severe Decompensation

During grief, a tendency exists to globalize conclusions and to fear a possible uncontrollable escalation of corresponding feelings. Yet, it is important to respect all feelings and to empathize with the person who experiences loss as a catastrophe. Whenever possible, the person is helped to understand feelings and to contain these feelings, under the umbrella of natural human responses.

The tricky part is to contain thoughts and feelings without minimizing someone else's experience. Going with the globalization can escalate feelings and increase rigid thinking. On the other hand, attempts to de-escalate feelings never work when the attempt may minimize the person's grief, sounding like condescension or phony empathy. Thus the most successful approach is to help the person understand that some grief responses are more complicated than others and some behaviors work better than others. This is a fact and not a judgment. A feeling exists. A thought occurs.

The rule of thumb is to open up or increase complexity when there is limited possibility for decompensation or dysfunctional response. When a high risk is evident the opposite is true: decrease complexity and narrow the focus. To increase complexity, reduce a conversation to specifics. Ask for details. Search for other feelings. Wonder about additional thoughts and beliefs. Introduce the notion that thoughts, feelings, and beliefs change, minute by minute, hour by hour, and over time.

Professional treatment and care responses always seek to increase self-esteem, and to limit primitive dysfunctional behavior that may be harmful. Specificity enlarges the grief story and empowers the person. Specificity also brings to light those aspects of the grief process that may be challenging and may lead to dysfunctional behavior. These responses might otherwise remain hidden and thus increase the power to do greater damage in the long run. Thus, through the specifics of an individual's experience, he or she moves through the various thoughts, feelings, and beliefs that will eventually build self and promote his or her unique form of recovery. Therefore, the person is encouraged to be as specific as possible. When appropriate, he or she is helped to complete the task of linking specific pieces of experience to create an even more complex picture that is truly more representative of the loss and grief.

Positive Strategies

- Encourage the use of everyone's correct name and the names of significant others involved in the loss.
- Encourage the use of direct statements and specific pronouns.
- Use open-ended statements and questions that narrow ambiguous expressions.
- Help the person use words to describe preferences, choices, beliefs, multiple thoughts, and multiple feelings.
- Seek out each story that goes with each exact experience.
- Ask for clarification of any term that is used even slightly differently than expected or customary. Note what is highlighted by tone or inference. Wonder about words that may have multiple meanings.
- Look for the gold mine of information that points to the core of who a person is.

STRATEGIES FOR DEVELOPING
A SENSE OF RELATIONSHIP

Since grief is an experience brought on by loss and separation, establishing connections with others is crucial. Just as it is important to cultivate a sense of self that is separate from that which is lost, so, too, is it important to validate connections whenever possible. However, validating continuing external connections is challenging. Even the most prepared person may not be able to handle the experience that often leaves even intense loneliness that sooner or later sets in after significant loss. This is true even when the loss does not involve death. Nonfinite losses (such as divorce, loss of custody of children, a major illness, experience of violence and other trauma) have a tendency to leave people feeling isolated even when surrounded by others.

Help the Person Fight Isolation

Clayton had worked for many years in the health care field as a nurse. When the media continued to cover the alleged pedophilia that had occurred over the past thirty years right there in his state, he was horrified. He was Roman Catholic and so was his mother. Her response was to tell him that they needed to stand behind their priests. He made no excuses for the priests. As health care provider, he was quite knowledgeable about pedophiles and the difficulty that this disorder presented in regard to effective treatment and recovery. Still, he found himself posing questions to a colleague that demonstrated his grief, "I just don't understand why the victims didn't speak up sooner." He had never considered how isolated a sexually abused victim feels. He had never considered how much power the church and the priest, in particular, has over the family. He had never thought of the denial that would face a good Catholic boy who went home to a good Catholic family and "told such lies about the Father." He also had never really understood how strong the denial mechanism is when tragedy occurs and how lonely that process can make a person feel. After the conversation with his colleague continued for a while, Clayton realized, "Now I understand why a class action lawsuit can be empowering to those who have been isolated in their grief and secrecy for so long."

Certain losses bring even greater experiences of isolation than might otherwise be found in normal grief responses. Some of these losses have been previously identified as complicating factors. The helper is often able to reach those who are feeling isolated by focusing on the person with caring and skilled attention to his or her experiences and needs. At the appropriate point (after the person has completely told his or her story) isolation needs to be named for what it is—an automatic attempt to protect self from further pain, injury, and grief. The typical thinking of a person who has experienced many losses and wishes to remain insulated, or isolated, is, "If I don't care about anyone, or anything, I won't get hurt again." The person attempts to deny the essence of his or her humanity, which is the striving to be connected to others.

One successful intervention is to gently ask what the person thinks his or her world would be like if he or she stopped caring. By extending a thought that is founded upon a fear to its extreme, the person may be able to see that caring is a value, or that the thought is unrealistic, and therefore, a distortion of what is humanly possible. An equally possible alternative is to go with the resistance and need for protection that brings about the process of isolation, and bless that experience. This strategy would be a reframing effort, wherein something that hurts is seen as a blessing. If this approach is used, the choice of what to consider as the blessing must be believable although just a bit surprising.

Trudy feels so alone that she spends all day in her room and cries herself to sleep at night. She barely makes it to loss and recovery group. In fact, she only comes because she has to attend this group or she can't go outside for a cigarette. Instead of directly talking about how much Trudy is isolating herself, and listening again to how lonely Trudy feels after the separation from her husband, her therapist tries a new approach. Today, the therapist notes once again that Trudy has been using the practice of isolation for a long time. She begins to wonder if this practice has moved from a normal protective response, to a complication, and perhaps has become a part of dysfunctional grief.

The therapist greets group members and proceeds to recognize Trudy's need for sleep and time alone. When Trudy intrudes on the therapist to say that she cried all night, the therapist takes a different tack and speaks with conviction about the blessing of tears. Tears, according to the therapist, are like a washing machine cleaning clothes: they wash away the grief. Trudy is encouraged to spend as much time as possible in bed and to cry as frequently as possible. Except for activities of daily living, and perhaps the loss and recovery group, she is encouraged to handle her grief in this preferred way. On most occasions, when the timing and approach is good, and the person needs to be urged to look differently at himself or herself, the person will say, "But, it isn't working for me. I feel more alone than ever, and I am exhausted from all this crying, so I am just caught in a vicious cycle." Either way, a person must, in the end, come to the realization that isolation may be helpful to a point, but, beyond that, it becomes a personal choice.

Positive Strategies

- Use the term "loneliness" to represent an inner feeling that may occur in any circumstance.

- Use the term "isolation" to represent an inner experience of withdrawing from others while in their midst, or otherwise.
- Teach the importance of alone time (and how to learn to manage it) and normalize times of loneliness.
- Help with the development of plans to recognize isolating behaviors.
- Help the person plan specific coping responses.
- Spend time uncovering the specific feelings and thoughts that led to the desire to isolate oneself. Isolating behaviors usually indicate pain, hurt, woundedness, or other factors such as depression or anxiety.

Help the Person Build Bridges from Past Experiences to New Relationships

Debbie needed a place to live. The only place that seemed reasonable was to live with her mother. Her mother was open to this option and expressed willingness to have Debbie move in upon leaving the hospital. At first, Debbie was relieved and excited to be leaving the hospital and going home. However, it was not long before she began to have concerns and doubts about the plan. She found herself getting irritable. She began to cry for seemingly no reason. Within a short while, she began to experience vivid memories of growing up with her mother. She could see her mother, stone drunk, yelling at her. She could feel the pain of being slammed against the wall while being told that she was not good. She found herself conflicted emotionally and knew her discharge was in jeopardy of being prolonged.

Debbie brought her feelings, thoughts, and memories to group. Here, she learned that she was grieving. The dysfunctional family behavior she had experienced as a child and as a young adult, now led to an experience of anticipatory grief concerning what could happen should she move in with her mother. Having learned about the stages of grief, and other losses that she had been working through, Debbie was not surprised to hear that her painful relationship with her mother was another loss that complicated her present situation.

By helping Debbie look at her relationship with her mother, over time she was able to grieve the past as well as remember some good times too. She was able to consider setting some limits on what she would and would not do to get discharged. She called her mother and talked about her fears and about her concerns that her mother might start drinking again. It was this call that opened new possibilities in the relationship. Because her mother had been sober for over a year and was going to alcoholics anonymous, she was able to be less defensive, and to hear Debbie's grief story. In fact, Debbie's mother had her own grief story to tell. This sharing of thoughts, feelings, and wishes for the future became a bridge to building a better relationship.

In some cases, the loss experienced is final and there may be no possibility to create a real relational bridge through the isolating experiences of loneliness and grief that are part of complicated grieving. Although a spiritual bridge and a memory bridge may be completed, the more concrete, physical bridge may be impossible. Even if a person cannot build relational connections with the lost object, person, or with that which is desired, the person must be gently taught to step into other relationships. Yet, the more complicated the grief, the more difficult it is to restore, repair, or build other relationships. However, recovery does depend of the restoration of a sense of relationship. Thus, the helper holds within himself or herself a crucial piece of wisdom. We are never alone in the universe. We just feel as if we are alone.

The bridge to being a person living fully in the world is built step by step. Important building blocks include experiencing that someone is concerned enough to listen, to care, and to help. This is why practical help consists of working on the problem that the individual identifies as important. This may be even more important to healing than working in the areas that are identified by other people.

Positive Strategies

- Use the helping relationship to build a reparative relational experience.
- Use the helping relationship to help build other relationships, i.e., bring in other family members and significant people, and help with referrals and consultations.
- Recognize and affirm ways that a person reaches out to others.
- Reframe talking, showing up, anger, and even silence, as ways of connecting with others. Make sure the reframe is plausible.

Witness to a Person's Grief

Connections come in many ways. Therefore, working with grieving individuals is a very humbling task that succeeds not only as the result of skill or of personal art. There is always a third factor that can be called mystery. If the working relationship is developing in a solid way, then there is room for the unexpected. In fact, the unexpected is a blessing when it occurs. Amazingly enough, this can be true even if the unexpected seems negative at first. Strategies that leave room for something new, unexpected, or different to happen are crucial in grief work.

In the summer of 1995 my family and I took an Alpine splendor tour. Two years previously my mother had died after four very difficult years of battling cancer. She had lived longer than expected. During those four extra years she changed her focus and began to develop a softer, more relational, side. She had always valued family but some of her ways of showing care for others did not always have the effect intended. Some relational bridges had in fact been badly damaged. Some were strong, affectively, but filled with painful experiences too. These issues were contained in the grief stories that the fifteen members of the family took with them as they traveled to Europe together.

The trip was fun. Relationships were made stronger. A new story was being forged moment by moment. Then came the unexpected. With it came insight, pain, and a grief that bridged the lives of strangers and human history. It connected our family with the larger pool of loss and grief that is part of the essence of life and part of its mystery.

The family stopped in Munich. Here, the tour guide offered to take whoever wished to go to Dachau. Dachau was a concentration camp during World War II. Dissidents, professors, Catholics, developmentally challenged, and Jewish people were some of those who died at Dachau. Upon arriving, we saw the pictures and read the stories. We walked the gravel paths and could look over the small brick wall and wonder why no one responded to what they clearly must have seen going on there. We saw the huge set of multiple train tracks that led captives from Munich to the camp. We stood in the remaining wooden buildings and could not imagine the number of people they had to contain. We looked at the platform with the gallows rope still hanging there. Then, we went around a little secluded corner and into a building with a shower room that would have looked like an ordinary group shower to those entering. From there, we went into the next room and saw the tiny furnaces intended to consume emaciated bodies. Finally, we went from one chapel to another that surrounded the back wall of the camp. Here, we prayed and we cried. In those two hours, we experienced firsthand the grief that we had only read about.

We left Dachau having been turned into authentic witnesses to our world's continuing grief. We thought of the people back home who still contend that none of this horror actually happened and we realized the importance of what we had seen and what we had experienced. Thus it is with anyone who connects with another's grief. True connections bring a crucial kind of intimacy and companionship that is a primary factor in all healing and transformation.

Being a witness to another person's grief does not actually mean walking the same path. This is an error brought on by a subtle denial mechanism that often happens during grief and is often transferred to the helping relationship. The form of this denial is often phrased to sound something like this: "If you have not been in my exact shoes you can have no idea of the grief I am going through." Although this rationalization sounds somewhat reasonable, its purpose is to defend against pain, intimacy, and fear.

It is helpful to remember the importance of a person's unique grief story and at the same time hold an awareness of the universality of loss and grief. A helpful response to the reverse plea for understanding is often a version of, "No, I do not fully understand your experience. Tell me, so that I can better understand." Implied in this response is the willingness to be a witness to the person and to the relationship that now exists, no matter how temporary, between helper and individual in need.

Positive Strategies

- Deflect comparisons of the magnitude of any individual's grief while accepting that some losses are truly horrific.
- Accept all grief and refrain from defending anything or anybody.
- Without too much self-disclosure, deflect some projection by indicating that trauma may have been part of many people's experience. Do this for a treatment purpose, such as building human connections, not for differentiation of self.

Strive to Mirror Experience and Help the Person Develop His or Her Own Vision

In the early stages of grief, the person experiencing the loss is able to tell just one grief story. This is a personal story and thus very powerful. It is important to restoration of self that the personal story be told. Early on, there is no room for the strategy of mirroring, or letting the person experience himself or herself at the moment. This would be experienced as another separation and would not be considered respectful. However, telling the grief story over and over is a way for the individual to build mirroring experience.

Witnessing to the grief story, and to what is happening within the person as he or she tells the story, has the effect of creating new experiences that are now shared in the present. Noticing how the grief story grows and changes, and how it stays fixed, are compassionate ways to companion a person in grief. When a person sees himself or herself more clearly, and is aware of being a complex individual, the mirror no longer needs to reflect what was or even what is. It can also provide a glimpse of the future. This is the stuff of hope and vision.

Just as a child is taught to see if his or her face is clean by using a mirror, so, too, does a person find the depths of grief, and the resources for transformation and recovery, by learning to listen to self, and becoming a witness to personal grief. When a therapist feels empathic to the grieving person, he or she is acting as a grieving person. When this empathy is expressed appropriately, the individual is given an opportunity to connect with and witness another's grief. For hope to emerge and healing to occur, this witness must become a vehicle for a genuine, and noncontrived mirroring experience.

It took a while for Rosemary to experience the power of mirroring for healing the wounds of grief. Rosemary hurt her child. She did not want to talk about it. In fact, she hid the fact from others. When they asked her if she had children, she hurt inside, and found ways to avoid the question. Her children were no longer under her care. She was young and had not been able to care for her children for a variety of reasons. She preferred to talk about what was happening during the day that she met with the therapist. She used the same approach in this group.

This went on for some time. Her grief story had no past, only a present. The group did not seem to notice. After all, they had their own grief to process. After months of this, Rosemary had built a solid picture of herself. In fact, the therapist began to wonder if what she was presenting was all there was to Rosemary. Maybe she didn't really cognitively understand or remember what had happened.

However, life is mysterious or perhaps just run by coincidence or fate. First, the men and then the women in the loss and recovery group began to talk about the painful abuse they had received from their parents and about their continued complicated lives and unfinished grief. Some members were challenged about whether they had been caring in their choices as it affected their children. The leader suggested that many parents don't have the skills to parent. Perhaps they didn't really know how to behave. Maybe they didn't have the capacity to love in a nonhurtful way. Needless to say, much division was evident in the group regarding that notion. After all, aren't people born with the natural talent of being able to love?

This kind of conversation went on session after session. Everything was framed at least once a session in terms of stages and processes of grief. A huge mirror was held up critically to parents and others who were not in the room. Sometimes, the mirror was turned back toward an individual. One could tell that Rosemary listened closely to all that was said. In fact, the leader was aware of thinking of Rosemary's history that Rosemary had not even disclosed privately with her.

One day, in a one-on-one session, Rosemary began the session angrily. She had paid for what she did. She knew she had done wrong. This was followed by further revelations in the next weeks. She had hurt her child. She felt guilty. She worried what the child would think of her when grown up. She realized that at the time she had been in an awful relationship where she was being abused. She had been very alone. She should have asked for help, but she didn't. From here on in, the mirror Rosemary held up had life and depth, even in pain. She had done two things. She had seen, from a safe position, the mirrors that others held up, and moved all over the place, in an effort to reflect reality. She noticed that no matter how bad the stories were, or how ugly the picture might be in the mirrors, everyone was treated respectfully. The group was hopeful while being realistic and leaving room for the present and the future.

Positive Strategies

- Consider how to feed back to the person what you experience about that person. Pay attention to appropriate timing. Adjust the feedback to just the amount that is likely to create moderate interest, or tension, between what the person is choosing to think or believe and what you observe.
- Consider yourself as a mirror that lends aspects of the self that the person may not see at this time, or may never have seen (such as hopefulness, courage, faithfulness, and other character attributes).
- In some cases, lend a mirror of anger, revenge, frustration, or desire. But, do so when it makes sense for a person to have these feelings or to have responded that way, even if it was not beneficial to the person.

Reach Out

Herb had been hospitalized a number of times in recent years. He was a good man, possessing great compassion and sensitivity. On his good days, he was personable, even charming. When he grasped a concept, he took to it like the proverbial duck to water. However, when Herb needed to be hospitalized it was due to clinical depression that consumed him. Even if he was assigned to therapeutic groups he was too depressed to attend. During these early days of hospitalization, he spent most of his time in his room on his bed. Even those he knew, respected, and normally found helpful could not reach him. During these times, he received medication and rested. He undertook only the barest of essential movement.

Then, one day Herb would be found sitting in a chair, awake, and out where others were going about their day. During these times, he attended the loss and recovery group. He knew a lot about the stages of grief and had worked through many losses. He could not seem to work through the loss of mental health. He just could not get past his sorrow about how depression made him feel and how it robbed him of connectedness with his family whom he loved dearly.

Complications such as a major or chronic illness make it difficult to reach out to those who want to be helpful. Often, direct prompting is needed. During these times, any work, whether physical, mental, emotional, social, or spiritual, needs to be presented concretely and simply. Priorities must be set stringently so that the person gets the essentials required for living. In this sense, the helper must figuratively reach out to the person in order to help. We understand this approach when dealing with a person recovering from surgery or one who is born with significant physical challenges. We need to realize that the person whose grief is severely complicated, and whose response is dysfunctional, needs similar help.

In inpatient settings, professionals, whose job it is to reach out, surround the severely impaired grieving person while that person is a patient. In the family and community setting, this strategy is often omitted. For outpatient services, an individual must contact and initiate most services within a fairly restricted framework. In families, concurrent grief processes often impair everyone's capacity to support a severely impaired person.

Reaching out and helping someone requires compassion and an intense desire to help another individual live a good life. This type of compassion is based on character principles of equity, justice, and altruism. It is always the therapist's job to reach out until the person says no, or is able to make another choice out of restored personal agency.

Positive Strategies

- Recognize that reaching out is your primary function.
- Convey that you are here to help the person.
- Indicate clearly when you can't help the person and refer in a delicate manner, for the person's benefit and well-being.
- Consider all situations where you feel that you are reaching out and the person is pulling back. It may be helpful to convey this experience in a nonjudgmental way and wonder how you might be otherwise helpful.
- Reflect and consult should you continue to reach out and the person responds by pulling back.

Use Your "Self" to Facilitate Treatment

Carolyn's response was a common one and the rest of the group supported it enthusiastically: "They don't care. They shouldn't work in a place like this if they can't be supportive." When asked who "they" were in her statement, Carolyn responded, "The staff, of course." As the conversation continued, it turned out that several employees were considered to be caring and supportive people. These people were supportive because they listened to the patients, answered questions, gave verbal and nonverbal feedback that indicated that they understood the patients' stress, respected their point of view, and tried to be helpful. The most common criteria for being considered a caring health care provider were listening, talking, and spending time with the person in need.

The use of self to facilitate treatment is not as intense a process as might be imagined by those who would prefer to be clinically more objective or aloof. Nor is the use of self a strategy intended to create a personal intimacy that is inappropriate for the helping relationship. Because losses are losses of connection, recovery is built on reorganization through the freeing of inner energy toward efforts at restoring connection or building new connections.

Second, because grief is a universal human condition, it is helpful to make use of connecting strategies that share the professional person's thoughts, feelings, and values in a generic sense. However, specific personal material that shares too much is not relevant to helping the person deal with grief. Too much personal material takes the focus away from the patient. A focus on self should be used only in the facilitation of treatment. The use of self for personal catharsis, personal processing of grief, chatting, or discharging any other function is not appropriate. Therefore, the professional use of self demands a rigorous inner questioning of helpfulness, appropriateness, desired outcome, and the capacity of the grieving individual to use the material offered.

Positive Strategies

- Put yourself in the person's shoes. Provide feedback about what you are trying to do when you model your experiences, thoughts, or feelings.
- When a person remains intensely angry with you about what you are or are not doing, accept these feelings and thoughts.
- On occasion, ask clients what they would do if they were in your position. This allows them to get closer to another person (you)

and enlarges their humanity and compassion. It also provides an opportunity for them to express their needs more clearly.
- Consider the therapeutic effects of sharing generic information and differentiate this from personal/intimate sharing. If in doubt, don't share. Never share for any purposes that are not clearly worked out before you speak.
- Make corrections when an intervention does not appear to benefit the grieving person.
- Stop in the middle of a statement if the intervention is not working.

STRATEGIES FOR CREATING
A SENSE OF MEANING

Since significant losses bring to light old and new questions of meaning, purpose, and connection, there is always a need to strategize how to incorporate these spiritual concerns. The one mistake commonly made by helpers is the failure to assess spiritual distress and grief. On the other hand, the way one addresses spiritual issues has a lot to do with whether one is helping or complicating the matter.

Facilitate the Building of Interior Containers
and the Development and Use of Helpful Rituals

The most straightforward and well-received intervention after the death of a loved one is the conversation about the rituals and services that family and friends are planning. Acknowledgment of barriers to planning and attending these events is crucial, as are any practical attempts to help the person determine which tasks are most important. Encouragement to attend some of the rituals is almost always a good idea, particularly if the person realizes that the intention of the ritual is to serve several functions. On one level, rituals are meant to relate to individual grief. On a second level, they are designed to relate to familial and intimate connectedness. On a third level, they promote communal grieving and healing. On all levels, the ritual is respectful to the deceased even though it is designed for the living.

To a certain degree, professionals fail to understand the several levels of connection provided for by rituals. When this is the case, they tend to leave decisions entirely up to the grieving individual. This is not without its costs because complicated recoveries frequently involve situations in which family, friends, and professionals have decided that it would be better not to go to a service or gathering. Often, this choice is not made from wisdom or insight, but from denial (fear, avoidance, unfinished business, rationalization). When alternative rituals are desired it may help if these rituals are undertaken for the purposes of personal grief rather than becoming a substitute for familial and communal grief.

Recently, there is a renewed interest in creating rituals to commemorate losses other than death. These public affirmations of a significant loss are often carried out at familial and small communal levels and are very helpful for grief recovery. This is true because a well-designed ritual is a container that is built to bear witness to all important life events.

Belinda benefited from the brief ritual of being escorted off the unit by her husband after undergoing heart surgery. She was fifty years old and the surgery had been successful. The operation and hospital time went all according to plan. Family, friends, and co-workers called, visited, and brought little gifts. The women at church and at her quilting guild organized a schedule of visitation, meals, and escorts to the hospital for blood work during the weeks that followed. Some friends planned to come regularly during the next four weeks to help Belinda with the walking program that was part of the follow-up care plan. Her pastor placed Belinda on the prayer list.

Each of these efforts was a care ritual that was set in motion to respond during this time. Belinda was aware of these efforts and she felt great comfort knowing that it was now her turn to be a recipient of this outpouring of care. She knew she was still in shock about the operation and probably a bit overwhelmed about the recovery period. She told herself that she was loved and supported, and that she could face the changes that might come in the next days.

Alex's experience was different. Before he was hospitalized in the psychiatric unit, he had been a successful carpenter. He had a spouse and children and was a regular churchgoer and a leader in the local Boy Scouts. Everyone in the community seemed to like Alex. He was always willing to lend a hand and had only good words to say about everybody. Then, one day he couldn't get out of bed. He didn't feel like getting up and told his wife to leave the shades down. He didn't go to work and didn't even call in to say he wasn't coming. He missed the church council meeting and didn't show up for the Boy Scout camping trip that was planned for the next weekend. He wasn't sick; he just didn't feel like doing anything.

By the second week, he was still not shaving and started drinking in the afternoon just to give him a boost. He skipped lunch and dinner and was irritable with the family. His wife told some of her friends that she was worried. When Alex's boss called, she didn't know what to say. Late one night after everyone was in bed, Alex got in his car and drove it into a telephone pole. He was taken to the hospital emergency room and five days later to the psychiatric unit. Even those who knew where he was did not call. No one knew what to do. As each week flowed into the next, people stopped talking about Alex and seemed uncomfortable. No one knew whether they should call, visit, or send a gift, so they didn't.

Alex was experiencing clinical depression and had admitted to attempting suicide. As Alex stayed in the hospital, his grief continued to deepen. No one came, even when he called and asked for visits. His wife only stayed briefly when she visited. The pastor did not visit, nor did he mention Alex's name from the pulpit during prayer concerns, out of fear that he might be breaking confidentiality.

Alex began to feel ashamed and guilty. He started to withdraw from family and friends. He didn't want to talk about what happened. He certainly wasn't going to accept that he had a mental illness. Nor was he going to tell anyone about his attempted suicide. When he was discharged there was no family gathering to welcome him home, no special meals, no thank-you prayer during the Sunday service, and no job. This was turning into an even bigger crisis than even he had imagined.

Three months later, Alex was hospitalized again. He talked about his losses and his feelings in recovery group. This time he was encouraged to learn everything he could about depression and its treatment. He made plans for rituals that would feel good to him when he was discharged. He thought of the meal he would make. He planned to watch a specific movie with the family. He called his new boss and explained what was happening and made arrangements for medical leave. He even called his pastor and asked to be placed on the prayer concern list. The group helped Alex anticipate future needs by processing the additional losses that had occurred after his last hospitalization. In this case, the planned events became little ordinary rituals that would give his life meaning and bring self-esteem and even small pleasures to his life. The main container he was building was the one that would declare that it was OK to have a major mental illness and it was OK to learn how to recover.

Positive Strategies

- Support generally accepted grief rituals, in their broadest sense, as being habits or practices that have helped many people during the early and acute stages of grief.
- Whenever you consider supporting the avoidance of customary rituals, consider whether this is unresolved grief on your part. Use your own resources to investigate this response within you.
- Clarify what is behind any desire to act without careful reflection. Ask what the ritual or new practice means to the person and to significant others.
- Facilitate the building of inner spaces as containers for the managing of grief and the development of meaning. For example, we have room for many feelings at the same time. We also have many beliefs.
- Seldom does one specific thought, feeling, or belief need to close out other thoughts and beliefs. As human beings we were created to be able to hold complexity. Holding rigidly to one thought, feeling, or belief to the denial of others that seem also to be present is a sign of dysfunction and usually requires grief therapy.
- Some useful inner containers are meditation, prayer, use of mantras, sitting still and noticing thoughts and feelings as they occur, imagining the soul or the core of being, developing an image of a safe place or a place to go at will.

Facilitate Mind, Body, and Spirit Connections

Meghan knew that grief was a natural process and that she was in the midst of it. She even knew that she was stuck in denial, anger, and sadness. It had been several years since she and her ex-husband had been given joint custody of her daughter. In reality, she was still the primary caregiver for her daughter, even though the ex-husband shared time with the daughter. Her daughter spent two weeks with Jeff every summer. In fact, the joint custody arrangement was going as well as could be expected, but, somehow, she couldn't seem to move past her grief. In her heart, she could not make the decision to move on from the failed marriage. It made no sense to her. She no longer needed to see a therapist. She had learned to practice meditative and thought-stopping techniques. She had learned to change her self-talk, to be more objective, and to be much easier on her self. Still, it made no sense to her. This she confided to her best friend who suggested that Meghan make an appointment with a pastoral therapist. Meghan felt she had nothing to lose.

Meghan met with Dr. Thomas and reviewed her loss history, temporary use of an antidepressant, and work with a psychologist who specialized in brief therapy. She seemed to know about the grief process and was able to indicate what her current thoughts and feelings were according to stages of grief. Her mind was quite sharp. She no longer needed antidepressant medication. She was eating well and sleeping a full eight hours. She had received a recent pay increase and was praised for her work in her last evaluation. She had even gone back to creating jewelry, which was a hobby started during her teenage years. Finally, she had met someone that she was growing fond of and the relationship was going smoothly at the moment. Still, the demise of the marriage made no sense to her.

The pastoral therapist asked about Meghan's religious and faith history. He inquired about her beliefs and paid particular attention to the beliefs she had held to since childhood. Meghan said that she believed in God and in the Bible. She had attended Sunday school as a child, been in the youth group, and even taken some courses on world religions during her college years. She ushered at church and was currently serving as a deaconess. Meghan believed in prayer. However, when asked if she currently prayed for herself, Meghan shook her head no. After all, what was the purpose for prayers now? This was the first time that Meghan had openly thought or talked about the faith crisis she continued to experience as a result of her divorce. She wasn't a religious fanatic, but just the questions and the encouragement to talk about the bigger picture was a relief to her. She felt a spark of energy growing.

Positive Strategies

- Become knowledgeable about the actions of mind, body, and spirit.
- Help the person identify how the actions of spirit connect with mind and body in his or her life, and vice versa.
- Recognize that all three realms (mind, body, spirit) are interconnected and can be under stress and change over time.
- Practice unconditional positive regard for the person's experience.
- Even when a professional assessment may contradict a person's understanding, be sure to ask what the person thinks, believes, experiences, or perceives of whatever is being discussed.

Affirm That Grief Work Is an Accomplishment

For many people, grief work seems like a waste of time, or even worse, indicative of a personal weakness. Until they learn otherwise, these beliefs about grief tend to complicate grief even more than necessary. To address the myths that surround the grieving process directly, a therapist will do well to refer to the grieving process as work. For those who have not heard grief described as work, this phrase comes as a surprise. A helpful response to such a surprise is to switch from intense feeling to momentary thinking processes. The thinking process further aides in opening a space for creativity in a context that seems temporarily safe.

Grief work is a phrase that provides dignity and significance to a very painful process. The fact that everyone needs to grieve adds a sense of commonality that can be supportive. The fact that everyone wishes that there was no such thing as loss and no need for grief further helps in learning about the importance of doing this task well. For most people, accomplishing a difficult task provides a sense of meaning. Recognizing accomplishments is a spiritually uplifting part of change and growth. Getting through tough times is often a badge of honor even if the outcome does not go as desired.

Harry didn't think he had to grieve anything. Life was awful from the beginning. He never really had it easy so it didn't do any good to talk about losses. So, he deflected every statement and focused on his daily agenda of things that must be done. Sure, he had lost his grandmother, but they weren't really that close. Yes, he had gotten in trouble for driving under the influence, but everyone he knew had that happen from time to time. His parents had separated when he was a child and he was no longer sure who his father was. Sometimes he had lots of energy and sometimes he didn't do much. That didn't mean he was bipolar. Harry wasn't openly negative, in fact, he kept his feelings guarded and was polite. He saw no reason for his referral to this loss and recovery group.

One day the group talked about how difficult it was to recover. Many members said they had been stuck in depression for years. They didn't think they could recover. They no longer knew what recovery looked like. They didn't think there was any reason for working on their grief. After all, didn't it just happen or not happen? When Harry contributed to the conversation the group leader took the opportunity to tell him what a hard worker he was and how much she was impressed by what she saw. Harry was clearly surprised. His face changed expression. The leader then went on to explain once more about the process of grief and why it was called work. She admitted that no one would want to take on grief voluntarily. She gave an example of a prominent person who had had significant loss and was quite specific about how that person had worked through grief. When the group was over, Harry walked to the door rather slowly. As he left, he very quietly said to the leader, "Thank you. No one seems to recognize how hard I'm working."

Positive Strategies

- Respect beliefs, thoughts, and feelings about grief while carefully inserting facts for consideration.
- Consider asking how the person learned to respond the way he or she does. Later, remind the person that much of what we rely on as adults we learned as children.
- When grief work is stalled with great affect, or noticeable absence of affect, shift to the here and now and work on issues in this arena first. When some relief occurs in the here and now, consider experiences that may have contributed to the problems in the here and now. Often this will circle back to an experience of loss.

Use the Term "Heart" When Referring to the Aspect
of Self That Makes Meaningful Changes

It could be said that recovery involves heartbreaking experiences and heart-making changes. This term, while more colloquial, has experiential meaning that corresponds directly to core responses within a person, while avoiding resistance that may be set up by the use of brain (thoughts), spirit, or soul, as seat for meaning. Let the person correct as needed. You will be beginning with a broad term that can be narrowed to provide a unique meaning for the individual.

The development of meaning is an internal as well as a relational process. Joel had yet to discover this fact. His wife, Virginia, knew that her marriage had lost its spark. She knew something was missing. Joel, however, had no idea what she was talking about. Everything seemed fine to him. They had a wonderful house and a camp at the lake. They had longtime friends and good jobs. Their children were happy and active in their own families. Now it was time for retirement, which they had planned for during the past ten years. They had imagined just what it would be like. But, now that retirement had come, their world seemed consumed by ordinary things that were boring. Three months after retirement, Virginia had a stroke. She had always had good health so this came as a surprise. Her left side was mildly paralyzed and no one knew if she would fully recover. Joel cared about Virginia, but he wasn't going to change what they had decided on so long ago. They'd just have to carry on with their plans.

Virginia came home slightly discouraged. She thought it over for about a month and then decided to visit her rabbi. They had a good talk. The rabbi assured her that he was not a marriage therapist. However, he thought she and Joel needed to discover what meaning life had for them as individuals, and as a couple, now that Virginia's health had changed. He suggested they go for couple therapy just to talk it out with someone objective. At first, Joel refused; he wasn't going to go to a shrink. After all, the stroke was just fate and he wasn't going to make a big thing out of it. Six months later Virginia had another stroke and it took quite a while for her to get her speech back. This drove Joel to action. Something was terribly wrong with the way their retirement was going. Perhaps he should get help. After looking all over the house for the therapist's name he finally found it and made the call. On the phone he found himself almost in tears and he blurted out, "This isn't fair."

The therapist was a woman. After listening to Joel she immediately had the image of a huge broken heart. At first, she thought maybe this would not be a good image for a man. She considered other approaches that might be more cognitive. She had no idea what his spiritual life was like and wasn't sure if she should talk about meaning so early in the process. Still, she had this persistent image of a broken heart. Several sessions went by and Joel told his story several times. He talked of what he had planned his marriage to be like. He talked of how he imagined retirement would be. Each time he got angrier and angrier. In desperation, the therapist finally blurted out passionately, "It sounds as though your heart is broken. You are thinking with your head. You are feeling from your gut, but it is your heart that is wounded. Let's talk about that."

At first, Joel was silent. He seemed taken aback by his therapist's words and her passion. He wasn't a mushy person and wasn't given to flowery words. But here in the safety of this room he felt a floodgate open. His heart *was* broken and he feared that no ray of sunlight or meaning would ever return.

Positive Strategies

- Recognize that important changes must come from internal motivation that makes sense, or is meaningful, to the person regardless of what others make of it.
- All conclusions are the responsibility of the individual. Your task is to facilitate the consideration of everything possible.
- Use concrete words with concrete people.
- Use sensate words with people who are more sensate.
- Do not use thinking words to talk about meaning. Use the term "belief" in its broadest connotation.
- When great intensity of feeling is evident, even negative feeling, consider the use of the term "passionate." It is more acceptable at times than rage.

State the Obvious: The First Step Is to Survive

In the past two decades, the term "survivor," has been used to refer to those who have had traumatic experiences of all kinds and are alive and even recovering from those experiences. Recently, some people have not wanted to be called survivors. The term is too public an announcement of what they have been experiencing as they have struggled to recover from significant loss. For some people, the meaning of survivor keeps them forever labeled by their traumatic experience. For these reasons, it may be wise to omit the term when helping people unless they prefer to use it.

However, the notion that being alive is a good thing is important to recovery. Complicated and dysfunctional grief responses always have the potential of becoming life threatening even if such a specific threat does not exist. This potential frightens people and frequently leads to concerns about life's multiple and rich meanings.

Survival is important. Other words that can be used refer to being alive, being safe, having connections, and accomplishing the seemingly impossible during the midst of horrendous events. Whether one uses the term survivor, exploration of that which gives life meaning is crucial to keeping alive the hope that causes a person to experience otherwise seemingly impossible times.

Positive Strategies

- Ask the person about his or her life, what it has been like, and how he or she has made it through.
- Recognize that survival is crucial and is an accomplishment in its own right, yet it may not result in quality of life. Rather, it is a first step.
- Develop specific behavioral plans for times when the person may not wish to survive or may have trouble doing so.
- Set limits on destructive behaviors and be prepared to follow through.

Affirm That There Is Life Beyond Survival and Hold That Fact for the Person Until He or She Can Grasp It

Meaning has no time line, but it has history, and it has implications for the present and for the future. However, because meaning is built on spiritual foundations, it can be dampened, lost, repressed, made obsolete, and be temporarily powerless when applied to life after significant and multiple losses. Yet these are not the whole story because there is a rhythm to life that gives us meaning. Sometimes, we go through brief periods of calm that are surrounded by horrible events.

Still, even in these times, it is possible to recover from each loss. In this sense, recovery is like a gift that keeps on giving. Every recovery brings growth, increased meaning, and a profound sense of connection. Every successful recovery makes life more than survival. It makes it an accomplishment!

In the beginning, Heidi felt guilty and did not believe that she had a clinical depression. She did everything she could to deny it. She invented other self-deprecating reasons for her loss of health. She would not listen to anyone. She told her story repeatedly and continued to suffer. When she was forced to take an antidepressant, her mood was a bit more stable, but she continued to believe that she did not have an illness. She stuck to her story that her experiences were the result of character flaw for which she alone was responsible. The medication helped her to be more patient with others and to listen despite her beliefs.

Months later, Heidi began to wonder if she could recover. Eventually, she gave a bit of credence to the possibility that she suffered from a clinical depression. She would occasionally declare that she felt more like herself on a given day. During this time, she began to end each session with the question, "Do you think I can recover?" She did recover, and for the time being needed to take medication. However, she no longer needed therapy. She focused on a life beyond her experience of hospitalization. She began to feel certain that there was life, despite a continuing mental illness.

Positive Strategies

- During the middle part of depression, help the person remember what it was like before the loss.
- During reorganization, help the person focus on times of gain and accomplishment.
- Encourage the support of others who are in recovery. This altruism and empathy builds hope.
- Help the person wish and fantasize what life would be like "if" it could be the way he or she wants it to be. Accept even dysfunctional responses. Explore these types of responses during reorganization as they may be remnants of denial brought about due to the challenges of making changes.

- Sometimes, change magical thinking into mystery and humbly acknowledge that the world can be surprising and amazing.

STRATEGIES FOR BUILDING MEMORIES

Look for the Beginnings of Memories

Every memory has a beginning and is the building block of one's life story. Some people collect memories and store them as treasures, whether painful or positive. Some memories come unbidden as is the case with posttraumatic stress memories. Other memories are consciously used again and again for purposes known, or unconscious, to the individual using the memory. All memories are powerful. This is why the loss of memory is so threatening to self and to loved ones. However, memories are not static energy and when they are treated as fixed elements they can make life rigid and dysfunctional.

In grief therapy, it is crucial to listen to one's memories through the medium of storytelling. It is equally crucial to explore the beginning of a memory. The beginnings of a memory set the stage for how the memory will grow and the service it will provide later on in an individual's life. Not every memory needs to be so meticulously investigated, but those that are brought to therapy should be treated as important data. Also important are those memories that should exist but don't seem to be presented in the grief process. Exploring the beginnings of memories sets the wider context for the meaning that a person will make of events and relationships.

Week after week, Darlene shared one story, based on one memory. The story was that her parents didn't love her and that nothing she ever did was right. She gave ample evidence of this lack of parental devotion, and of the effect it had on her current relationships, and the struggle that brought her to therapy. She knew that she was stuck in anger that alternated with depression. The amazing thing to her was that she could help others but she couldn't help herself.

Six weeks into group therapy, Darlene was asked what caused her to believe that her parents never loved her. She provided plentiful evidence that supported her belief just as she had in the past. This time, the therapist made no response to these stories. When Darlene came to the end of her painful litany of truly traumatic experiences, the therapist asked her to remember the first time she knew she was not wanted or loved. Instead of accepting a quick defensive answer, the therapist assured Darlene that there was plenty of time, and that the group would wait while she thought through her response. The group concurred. Everyone sat silently. After five minutes that seemed to go on forever, Darlene had an answer.

She remembered a time she had stood behind the living room door. She was trying to peek into the room to see what kind of mood her parents were in so that she could decide if it was safe to come into the room. She was fourteen years old when she heard her drunken mother say to her equally inebriated father, "I wish Darlene had never been born." Then, she heard her father's slurred voice say, "That girl has never been anything but a disappointment." Now, it made sense. Everyone in the group remembered that these were the exact words that Darlene currently applied to her own life.

Positive Strategies

- Look for memories beneath memories.
- Ask for first memories of many thoughts, beliefs, feelings, and experiences.
- Explore repetitious memories, powerful memories, and dream memories.
- Note where memories are lacking or incomplete, or perhaps do not make sense.
- Teach the idea that memory comes from somewhere, is stored somewhere. It is activated in some way and influences us somehow. In this sense it is never static. For the purposes of recovery, it is helpful to learn how memory works in each person's case.

Recognize and Help with Unbearable Memories

Sometimes, unbearable memories must be recognized, placed in a tightly sealed box, and put in mental storage for however long the memory is overwhelmingly active. Paradoxically, boxing the unbearable is sometimes the only way to make it bearable and keep the memory contained. It is crucial that the grieving person and the helper understand this fact about some memories. If a memory cannot be a helpful part of one's life, it cannot be allowed to continue to be overwhelmingly hurtful. This acceptance means that not every experience can be reasoned out, analyzed, or have energy discharged from it. Sometimes, nothing can be gained from a negatively charged horrific memory. When this is the case, it needs to be deactivated. Continuing to try to make sense out of some horrific events gives them more energy. Thus there is a time to explore memories and there is a time to let them be within an inner safe containment field.

Positive Strategies

- Some memories are unbearable even in the midst of bearing them. This is a fundamental paradox of horrendous memory and traumatic loss that needs to be recognized.
- Some events have no reason or make no sense that is acceptable to a person, so our job is to help that person carry the memory.
- Help the person find a community (or one other person) in which to share the burden of the unbearable. This is when self-help groups may be a blessing.
- Affirming the unbearable can give the person permission to recover.
- Suggest that the person develop practices for letting what has been, be, because it cannot be changed.
- Help provide models/mirrors of people who have experienced the unbearable and survived.
- Help the person to know that help is available until the person is able to bear the memory.
- Suggest thought-stopping techniques, not for the purpose of suppression or denial, but for the purpose of managing memories and working on them during more stable and safer times.
- Develop and promote a "first things first" attitude and cycle of interaction. Safety first, functioning next, processing the memory comes afterward.

Help the Person Make Meaning Out of Memory

The meanings we gain from memory are not always pleasant, but they can still be insightful. When exploring these meanings, it is always important to explore the process by which meaning is gained. Memory always gets carried forward for a reason.

Kim's memory was crucial to her decision that birthdays were important to her. In her family, everyone always makes a big deal about having a birthday party on the day of the birthday. When Kim was thinking of a friend whose spouse just came home from a major heart surgery that had included a postsurgery infection, she wondered if there would be a birthday party five days later on his birthday. The person recovering from heart surgery apparently liked to have a big celebration on his birthday.

Kim felt that it was essential to her for her adult children to have a big party for her on her birthday, so she understood that this man would want the same thing. When challenged to consider how important this would be, given the timing and vulnerability of his health situation, Kim stood firm. She stated that when her mother was dying and did not want to eat any longer she had not fed her, even though her sister had protested. When her dad had been facing death, he had insisted that all of his children and family be there with him. So, Kim thought that if the guy wanted a birthday party five days after his open-heart surgery and postinfection, then that was up to him.

The only complicating fact that nagged at Kim's friend, who was also a grief therapist, was the small fact that there was no reason for this man to be treated as though he was near death. He had just had the surgery so that his life wouldn't be compromised and so that he wouldn't die. The question the therapist-friend mumbled was, "Is it true that what matters is only what an individual wants, or do relational issues also matter?"

This conversation continued off an on throughout the week. There was ample opportunity to talk through the changing events of life and the need for adaptability. There was time given to the inner recognition of each one's values and needs. Meanwhile, Kim gave the man's spouse several ideas about how to manage the birthday. She was pleased, for his spouse was very grateful to have these suggested options.

Positive Strategies

- Ask, "What does that memory mean to you?"
- Wonder why a memory comes and goes at specific times.
- Wonder what may be implied behind the memory.

Help People Edit Their Own Stories

It is common for people to think that life is written in stone. Seldom do people think they can affect the past, even if they feel more optimistic about the present and the future. Although it is true that even the last moment is technically gone, it is still open to possibility through the process of memory and the externalization of meaning. In this way, one can affect one's own past story and memory, and actively decide how to carry each into the future. People do change their feelings over time. They change their perspective and they gain new information and insight. This is the reason why therapy is such an effective tool for change.

For example, a young man initiated one of the most exciting moments in group therapy. His own life story was dreadful. This session, a room full of women who had severe trauma histories became too much for him. Time and again, the women would tell the truth of their experiences, never wavering in their pain and grief. The story never changed. No new information was added. No new perspective was introduced, no change in tone of feelings. Even though Henry was struggling with his own helplessness and depression, he found himself saying, "It's your story. You can change it any way you want to change it." The thought was stunning. Its objective truth was not important, for to a certain degree, there is no objective truth. From there on, everyone thought about how they would like to edit their stories. Once the possibility existed, they took seriously what it might mean to make changes. Just the freedom to edit memories was powerful, suggesting the possibility of moving on to reorganization and recovery.

Positive Strategies

- After a relationship has been built, broaden loss and grief to include the term "grief story." Explain that story does not mean fictional, but rather to experience having beginnings, middles, and endings.
- Notice changes that are added to the story.
- Have the person imagine any recovery endings that might be possible.
- In group settings, encourage others to talk about changes that they have noticed in their memories and grief process over time.

- Help people select memories that they would like to cherish.
- Help the person understand that intrusive memories can also change over time and with professional help. Offer this as hope rather than promise.

STRATEGIES FOR RECOGNIZING
CONTINUITY OF BEING

The spiritual dimension of the grieving individual must keep pace with the other dimensions engaged in the grief process. For it is through the spiritual dimension that one experiences the wholeness of existence, or complete healing, and recovery. Meaning, purpose, and connection must be embraced anew on a regular basis. However, this spiritual fact must be reformulated thoroughly after every significant loss. The phrase "continuity of being" is used to describe this meaningful sense of self as deeply connected and committed to life. For a deep commitment to life, one must intimately experience deeper and deeper connections to meaning that transcends oneself and all one knows. This is essential, for it is never possible to know all about the truly meaningful aspects of life. Significant loss, and the consequent grief, sneaks up on spiritual reality like the shadow in the night that says, "You do not know me, but I am here."

Help the Person Embrace Mystery

Embracing mystery is one strategy for resolving grief. Once we are through sorting and sifting all that we know, or think we know, about our relationships, we must accept the fact that we actually know very little. Thus, each loss is an opportunity for humility, for celebration of what was, and for what is and will be.

In the Old Testament, God declares the ultimate mystery in the definition of God, "I am who I am" or "I am what I cause to be." So, too, is this the essence of all of life. The lost object, person, or dream, is forever what it is, whether past, present, or future tense. We human beings are who we are. This is the mystery of past, present, and future. It is the ground of existence, or continuity of our being, and of all being. In this sense, gain and loss, pleasure and pain, and all other opposites, are forever united in the mystery of life that we must nod to as part of the condition of living.

It is a skill and an art to embrace mystery as life, to walk on paths that are clear, and travel ways that are known. It is also an art and a skill to embrace mystery as life and walk in places where no paths exist, travel ways that surprise us, having no sense of where we will be tomorrow. Mystery's basic tool is represented by helplessness on the one hand and by hope on the other.

Positive Strategies

- Insert the concept that what we know and don't know changes over time.
- Normalize the desire that all of us have to control our lives.
- Recognize times we have been able to control something and it has worked for us, and times when that controlling effort has not had predictable, or positive, consequences.
- Focus on developing hopeful practices for living with mystery.

Lift Up Healing Moments

Healing moments are those times when we experience the mystery of feeling better connected with who we are and what life is all about. We experience our version of personal, intimate, and transcendent spirit. These healing moments are part of the mystery of life.

Unfortunately, or maybe fortunately, we seem to experience healing most profoundly after fragmentation, illness, disconnection, or other diseases and distresses that bring on the grief process. Each part of the human dimension has its own distress that leads to healing moments. Physical and mental illness is acutely felt through symptoms and behaviors that lead to fragmentation that must be addressed for healing to occur. If no interventions occur the illness will continue, and in most cases, will cause the destruction or demise of the person. This is also true of emotional, intellectual, social, and spiritual distress. That which brings about a healing moment can only be realized in a limited way. It is true that we can build up a resource of experiences, and learning from those experiences, that can be applied in similar cases of illness and distress. It is not true that every person will experience healing by applying similar resources. Thus, we return to the mystery of life. This is the temporary truth about healing.

Healing happens. It does not always happen in the same dimension as the fragmentation. It can be helped and it can be hindered. But, healing cannot, with absolute certainty, be directed.

Positive Strategies

- Help people increase their awareness of healing moments.
- Strive to increase your awareness of healing moments.
- Help promote the identification of healing moments within one's larger environment.
- Help people remember healing moments.
- Pray for healing moments.
- Set yourself in a position to receive healing.
- Practice acts of gratitude.
- Share experiences of amazement.

EXPRESSING GRIEF IN OTHER WAYS

Grief must be expressed. It must move and flow. Some of its movement is internal. Some of its movement is related to a higher spirit. Some of its movement is connected to others. Although talking about grief has tremendous benefits, and promotes recovery, it is often important to supplement this approach, or even substitute this approach, with other mediums. The choice of expressive medium is predicated by the preferences and needs of each individual. Journaling, craft or hand therapy, expressive movement, and engagement of the imagination are four expressive techniques that have been particularly successful in the productive expression of grief.

Journaling

Journaling has become a strong therapeutic tool in the popular as well as clinical realms. The use of journaling specifically for grief therapy is appropriate. Journaling is of particular benefit during the depressive and reorganization stages. During the early stages of grief, the task of journaling can inhibit the unsorted jumble of feelings and thoughts that are essential to the process. Exceptions to this would be in cases of chronic complicated grief. When grief about multiple and traumatic losses has been in process for a long time, it can also be helpful to write about problematic feelings, thoughts, and behaviors that are strongly held. Common, large, spiral notebooks are best for this activity. It is helpful to do a loss history on a chronological timeline. An extended loss history, through up to three generations, is helpful for situations in which multiple and inherited generational losses have occured. Persons can be taught to do assessment of the stage (or stages) of grief that they feel describes where they are on any given day. Directed reflection assignments can also be part of journaling activity. By observing the person's response when journaling is suggested, one can assess whether a person is amenable to this activity. Both genders may be open to journaling, although experience indicates that more women respond to this during times of crisis. However, once a male has some success in journaling, the rewards are often great.

Craft or Hand Therapy

Craft or hand therapy is also a useful tool for those for whom words are not enough. This intervention can be part of classical grief therapy when it is used as an adjunct tool. It is true that some personality types need to work out their grief by means other than talking. In some instances, the type of therapy will be dictated by its simplicity and by a person's ability to incorporate grieving stories within the medium. However, any craft can serve to contain grief and to give it measured expression. For those whose grief is overwhelming, and who are prone to dysfunctional behavior, it is important to choose a safe craft such as drawing, working with clay, or stamping with rubber stamps. Once a person is safe, most other mediums are helpful. Some people sew, crochet, or knit. Others create pictures or quilts depicting losses and connections, or do woodworking. Most people benefit from therapy that focuses on reorganization and helps them reach into the future.

Vareen was in her middle years when she took up working with clay. She was an intelligent professional woman who had no hobbies. She was a hard worker who took no time to play. The death of Vareen's mother hit her hard.

She felt adrift. Life had made sense to her prior to her mother's death. Her work week was a mere forty hours. As her mother often said, she was lucky to have a job that she could do by the clock. At home she had the dinner on the table at six and spent the evening straightening the house and doing weekday chores. She was in bed by eleven o'clock. On weekends she did the real cleaning and the errands essential to a busy household. She did take time off to go to the baseball games that her husband enjoyed. She even joined him on his fishing trips, though she felt idle and restless.

A year after her mother's death, her therapist suggested that Vareen take up a hobby. Vareen was polite, but not enthusiastic. Several weeks later, the therapist asked her what she thought of the suggestion. Vareen rubbed her hands together in an agitated manner, looked at her lap, and quietly declared that her mother would not like it. As is so often the case, this experience was an opportunity to continue the grief process that had been temporarily stalled.

Two months later, Vareen came to therapy announcing that she was ready to learn a hobby. She asked the therapist which hobby would be good for her. The therapist avoided moving into the surrogate mother trap by declaring that the choice to learn a hobby was entirely up to Vareen. She could take up a hobby or not; the choice was hers. Vareen tried painting on wood, cross stitch, jewelry making, stamping, quilting, and leaded glass before she settled on knitting. Years later, she realized that she was not an outstanding knitter. But, she had made forty-eight afghans, and it was so relaxing, she started giving them to the local nursing home. She really could make sense out of life when she had those needles in her hands.

Movement

Movement, in general, is helpful to recovery. It is particularly helpful to those who experience depression. In these cases, exercise, cleaning, and gardening can be recommended as ways to increase well-being. For those whose thoughts are racing too fast, movement can be combined with listening to music for a calming effect. Therapists are cautioned to be realistic about strenuous exercise and to assess possibilities for dysfunctional use of this kind of movement. Referrals to a medical doctor or a physical therapist are often in order.

Milder forms of movement are just as beneficial in instances of grief. Here, the focus is on changing position. For those who are agitated, angry, and are likely to express that frustration or rage, large body movements need to be channeled into walking or into smaller body movements. Helpful smaller movements, such as getting up, shifting position in a chair, moving to a different part of the room, walking in one's own garden, getting a glass of water, can be amazingly reassuring to those who have difficulty moving at all, and to those whose movements must be contained.

Imagination

Imagination is a powerful tool. Creating and responding to the work of the imagination is often helpful to recovery. Often, the imagination is approached through symbols, internal and external images, pictures, and poetry. When grief is complicated or acute, imagination tends to be self-protective by being overly optimistic or profoundly pessimistic. Sometimes, imagination can be a safe way to express what cannot be expressed directly.

Jean was not particularly imaginative and she certainly didn't feel creative. She thought of herself as a practical and straightforward person. She knew she had an anger problem, but it was legitimate from her perspective. After all, the past two years had been just one loss after another. She was a good listener and attended group regularly. In fact, she never missed the loss and recovery group. She liked the leader and found her helpful. She learned the stages of grieving and could use this new language to process her thoughts and feelings. However, whenever any milestone came up she would tell the group that "if such and such didn't happen" she was likely to go ballistic.

This approach happened several times before Jean announced that her birthday was coming soon, and if she weren't out of the hospital by then, she would blow her top. This time, the leader asked her what she meant when she said that. Jean changed her words to, "I'll lose control." The leader asked what that would look like. Jean said, "I'll punch the wall and scream." Jean was told that she couldn't punch the wall, but if she wanted to scream it would be all right. The group agreed.

Jean chose not to scream. So the leader inquired about Jean's reasoning behind making these kinds of pronouncements. All the time, the leader was thinking that this was probably a way of making threats and part of an aggressive behavior pattern when things didn't go Jean's way. Although this may have been true, Jean's response was more insightful. She started to cry and said, "I've been away from home my last two birthdays and I want to be home for this one." Jean was able to share her fears, her loss, and her pain. The leader and the group supported her and told her that she could say that it hurt to be away from home on her birthday and that she hoped this year would be different. It was natural for her to be worried and to be anticipating the possibility of more grief in the near future.

TURNING AROUND UNHELPFUL GRIEF RESPONSES

It is possible to contend that the pastoral psychotherapist, or any therapist, comes more in contact with complicated and dysfunctional grieving than with normal, less complicated, responses. Since this may be true, the best resource that a therapist can provide for other helpers and health care providers is the perspective of being able to differentiate between intensity of grief responses and their productivity in leading toward grief resolution. Unproductive grief responses are those that create obstacles that require amelioration for grief to continue to a natural and healing resolution. In this category, there are responses that are not helpful and responses that are damaging. There are also responses that require reparative or restorative work. Ideally, it would be wonderful if grief work could be preventative, as with other stress responses, but this is not completely the case. However, education and supportive resources can assist people in striving toward normal, albeit painful, grief responses.

Unhelpful Responses

Unhelpful responses are any responses that promote destructive denial; collude with strong feelings to promote destructive behavior; accept any feeling, including sadness and sorrow, as a permanent condition prior to the sorting through of the relationship; encourages helplessness rather motivation to survive; and does not apply to skill deficits needed for reorganization or recovery. Unhelpful responses can come from any direction—internally, environmentally, or relationally.

Positive Strategies

- Set some limits on acceptable responses in therapeutic/helping situations. For example, talking is OK but acting on thoughts, feelings, and behaviors in the therapeutic/helping relationship is not OK unless negotiated under safe and therapeutic circumstances.
- Stop all risky behavior immediately.
- Help the person practice acceptable responses that affirm self, feelings, and needs.
- Teach choice and consequences in natural, straightforward ways.

Damage Control

Damage control refers to any strategy whose aim is to stop unhelpful responses. In a sense, most behavior therapy is damage control. In some cases, the damage or unhelpful response must be contained. In these cases, damage control is the equivalent of a big stop sign.

Barbara was hospitalized several times during her teen years. On her most recent hospitalization, she was very depressed and suicidal. Any change at all brought about the experience of loss and profound overwhelming grief. Clinical depression complicated her recovery from multiple and traumatic losses. Barbara's response was unpredictable, except for the fact that she continuously tried to kill herself. For this reason, she was placed on a visual precautionary level. This precaution was necessary for some time before any attempts could be made at dealing with her grief issues. Since she could not stop herself, others needed to do so on her behalf.

Jeanette's grief response also required a strong intervention from her family to help control her declining health situation. In her case, she was grieving the death of her husband of two years. Jeanette's husband had died in a military action overseas. Jeanette was pregnant when her husband died and so distraught that she did not take care of herself or the unborn child. Her family understood for a while, but then they noticed that she had lost a lot of weight. When they asked her how her pregnancy checkups were going, and if they could do anything to help, she said she was fine, and that she didn't need to see the doctor. This was when the family became aware that some damage control had to happen for grief to get back on track and for Jeanette and her unborn child to be safe.

Positive Strategies

- Consider if reparative work is possible and leave the choice and responsibility to the person.
- Help the person plan for future situations.
- Accept the reality that a person may have done something horrific and traumatizing to another person. He or she may have to live with that knowledge.
- Help the person recognize that the past is not the present, nor the future.

Reparative Work

Reparative work is probably best described as therapeutic efforts to assist an individual in the task of grieving more normally, and, if possible, unassisted by professionals. Reparative work usually involves the restoring of numerous processes to healthy functioning. Reparative work is often necessary when losses are traumatic, horrific, or there are multiple losses of significant magnitude. Reparations may need to occur throughout the various levels of human needs, or in some cases, reparations may appear to be confined to one area, but really affect several areas.

Positive Strategies

- Stick to the principle that, except in the immediacy of required action, all else is subject to inner reflection and insight before outer action is taken. Think, feel, believe, sort, and plan before engaging in the repair of relationships.
- Refer when necessary. Be caring and firm about the referral. Provide a clear explanation of the thinking process used to arrive at the referral decision.
- Report what needs to be reported. Tell the person that you need to do so and let the person express feelings and do what he or she needs to do.

SUMMARY

Much of grief work is experiential and even experimental. As with any other therapeutic and caring intervention, standards and strategies are available, but the true art of providing help is in the application and development of effective strategies. To this end, every helper is encouraged to keep good notes of strategies and their outcomes. To be honest, I wish I had done more of this over the past twenty-five years. It would have been helpful to have a record of the many interventions that did not work, the ones that worked miraculously, and the ones that took time for their impact to be discerned. At present, I have my memories, and some documentation that relate to specific cases, but my grief is that I learned this other approach the hard way. My advice is go with what you know as a professional, read and resource other ideas, and keep new interventions simple and respectful in all cases. Yet, the most important strategy remains the development of a habit of being authentic and connected to self and others. If the person you help gets just this one experience the person will be in a better place as a result of having been with you, no matter how briefly.

Chapter 8

Reorganization and Reclaiming One's Life

I hope to God you will not ask me to go to any other country except my own.

Chief Barboncito, 1868, p. 5

We sit in silence in the small rectangle of a room. Outside, the January deep freeze has covered everything, blanketing the world in white and winter gray. Inside, the four men and two women sit, brought together under the therapeutic theme of loss and recovery. The newcomer starts by saying that it is too much to talk about his losses. He goes on to mention a loss of placement in a program he had enjoyed for years. He then speaks of an extremely debilitating physical disease that will most assuredly lead to an early death. I can't tell his age. He may be twenty-eight or thirty. In any case, he is young. The person to his right, a teenager grown much too wise and weighed down for his young years says, "I can identify." He speaks of his physical problem, which may also lead to a very early death if something can't be done. In any case, he must change his lifestyle. The woman comes in so softly that I have to lean closer, even though I am sitting right next to her. She talks of a childhood disease that seems to have left a residue that returns in a mild form, under stress, and is aggravated when she is depressed. The room is silent, so silent that I imagine that the outside cold has oozed through the walls and left its grayness settled over all. I ask the forth person if he has had any similar experiences. "Oh, yes," he declares with heaviness of tone and words. Again we sink into silence. This time, the silence seems like a completed circle that binds us in our humanity, and in so doing, we do not rush to push it away.

Several minutes later, I try to use this moment of connection to wonder what can be helpful. The conversation flows with thoughts and ideas. There is a need for specialized resources and people you can trust. The desire is expressed for people in the medical field to do their jobs, run their tests, and draw blood with skill and compassion. A consensus forms around the notion that reorganization and recovery depend a great deal on personal responsibility, but recovery is also greatly enhanced by the manner in which professionals demonstrate their relational skills while doing what needs to be done.

REORGANIZATION INVOLVES CHANGE

In many cases, facing the change brought about by significant loss can feel as though one, like the Navajo Chief Barboncito (in the beginning quote of this chapter), is being sent to another country. Few go willingly. Most are overwhelmed by fears about what will await them, in that new place, without the significant relationship, dream, or object that had been so dear and central to them. No matter how frequently we experience loss, we wonder equally profoundly about change. Of course, some take to change better than others. So much depends on past experiences and on current resources.

Change is one of the most significant challenges that must be addressed during reorganization. Although change follows all losses, significant loss brings even more significant changes. In many cases, loss brings a continuous flow of change that happens throughout the grieving process. Plus, change often ebbs and flows with a fairly independent rhythm, with responses that are idiosyncratic to each individual. Thus, the process can seem to have a life of its own and requires a significant amount of energy, as well as focused resources. By the time a person is ready to reorganize, he or she is often drained and emotionally fed up with all of these changes and wants only to return to some sort of stability.

It is this search for stability that provides the energy needed to reorganize during most normal grieving processes. However, in complicated and dysfunctional grief responses there is often a lingering struggle to deny and resist change throughout the recovery process. For these people, reorganization continues to be a dreaded part of the whole process. In fact, change is so dreaded that many people choose to remain angry or depressed, rather than do that which is needed to reorganize.

Nevertheless, change is the central task of this phase. This is the part of grief that requires more action and initiative than the more reactive responses of earlier stages. This is emotionally true because changes, after a significant loss, seem new. One can never be the way one was before the loss. For this reason, the most helpful thing to share with a person, on the precipice of reorganization, is that it makes sense for them to be patient with themselves when making these necessary changes. Learning takes time. It is an additional burden to expect to be able to make changes quickly, smoothly, or even gracefully. Change takes time and follows its own process.

In *Changing for Good: The Revolutionary Program That Explains the Six Stages of Change and Teaches You How to Free Yourself from Bad Habits,* James Prochaska and colleagues (1994) list the following stages of change.

1. Precontemplation
2. Contemplation
3. Preparation
4. Action
5. Maintenance
6. Termination

This model of change does work well with the model of grief being presented, but it is important to remember that grief recovery (termination or the completion of a process of change) occurs in a somewhat circular system that has developing depth each time the process has occurred. It is not so much that one is partially recovered, or completely finished with a change, but, rather, one completes a change that then becomes part of another change. A bad habit may be terminated. But significant and meaningful attachments are a part of who we are forever.

In the following poem, "The First Time I Grieved My Father," the continuing change process is demonstrated. The poem refers to an incident in my childhood. It comes back to me, in this format, a year after my father's death. By this time, there were many years of reflection, new experiences, and even new information available as resources for the processing that is lifted up in this piece of poetry. The grief work surrounding my relationship with my father has been complicated. There were many large and small losses, as well as gains, over the many years before and after his death. Just one piece of information, provided by my birth mother many years before, now fit for the first time with emotional truth and spirit-filled satisfaction.

THE FIRST TIME I GRIEVED MY FATHER

I am small and dressed in flannel.
    The halls are barely lit and there are
    bars. It must be a crib, or something
    quite restraining, and I alone, so all alone.

I could have been two or up to six.
    The fishing done, the bark long peeled,
    the chickens hovering and last cards played.
    "That was the time your dad went to Texas,"
    my mother said. I didn't know.

And I was lost, and I was grieving,
    throwing up and running a temperature,
    "So much so that you had to be hospitalized
    for a month," she said. I didn't know.

They really didn't know what was going on
    but some thirty-two or more years later,
    my mother said, her insight clearing,
    "I guess you were upset
    at your father's leaving."

Profound internal truth is contained in the simplistic phrase, "everyone experiences loss sometime." Everyone grieves and suffers the sorrow of loss. It is also possible that during reorganization we must face an even larger cosmic truth. Beginning with birth, much of our life is a process of grieving. This is not said in a negative sense so much as a reflection of the care, connections, and passion that is so integral to life itself.

Because most losses bring about a grief process that tends to lead to change and recovery, it is doubly important to discover why a natural process is not always so natural and requires intense assistance. In working with complicated and dysfunctional grief responses, it is of vital importance to know what makes the difference between one person's recovery and the failure to recover that is the experience of others. Although I don't admit to having completely satisfactory answers, I have decided that certain types of motivators bring about more change and reorganization than others. So, I tend to focus on these motivators in situations in which people are stuck in denial, negative feelings, and depressive sorrow.

MOTIVATORS

In a prayer written by Thomas Merton (1990, p. 83), Merton says to God,

> I have no idea where I am going. I do not see the road ahead of me. I cannot know for certain where it will end . . . and the fact I think I am doing your will does not mean that I am actually doing so.

The most important therapeutic question in working with complicated and dysfunctional grief responses, next to safety and daily functioning, is the question of what will motivate a person to move from the earlier stages of grief to the latter stages of reorganization and recovery. For Thomas Merton, one could conclude that faith would lead him to walk forward, even though he cannot see the road ahead of him, and doesn't know if his movement is something that he should be doing.

Yet, all of us must move from our sorrows and begin sifting, or sorting, through our lost relationships. Once this is accomplished sufficiently (although not necessarily completely), then we must make an inner decision to keep going, to move on, and to recover. This truly becomes the faith part of the journey.

After paying close attention to the processes of those whose grief is complicated, I have noted five common motivators that tend to cause an individual to begin to reorganize his or her life after significant loss. These motivators are based on spiritual, religious-spiritual, social, relational, and time and healing factors. These factors tend to motivate those who have sorrowed a long time, and are exhausted, and those who have mulled through the lost relationship to the point that even they know they are ruminating with no new insight. However, an intervention to discern what will motivate a specific individual to reorganize his or her life is usually not appropriate during the early stages of acute grieving. Nor is such an intervention appropriate when an individual is in deep denial or dangerously angry. At these times, safety and daily functioning continue to be of prime concern.

Religious-Spiritual Motivators

Many individuals who do not currently attend religious services have been connected with a religious tradition during their formative years. When this is the case, they may be motivated to make changes in their life because of what they have learned from sacred scriptures and practices. For this reason, it is always best to ask individuals to talk about any beliefs they have, that are supportive, or that are of concern, at any time during the grieving process. This leaves the direction of inquiry open and appropriately respectful to differing practices and traditions.

However, in some cases, it is helpful to have an example of some belief motivators ready for the purposes of modeling responses that some people might have to the question. Be aware that some sacred writings will be quoted to justify wrath, rage, violent action, and revenge. If this is the case, then these writings and beliefs need to be explored by encouraging the individual to share thoughts, meanings, and applications that these statements have for them. After listening, it is possible to gently wonder if these truths apply, and if so, to what degree. An even better approach would be to accept these beliefs and ask if there are other beliefs that relate to finding peace, forgiveness, moving on, and turning unfinished grief over to a Higher Power or to God.

Four of my favorite motivational quotes suitable for Jewish and Christian traditions are from Psalms, Ecclesiastes, and Isaiah. I do not give these to the grieving person unless the person is unable to resource one for him or herself and the need is spiritually, and therapeutically great.

PSALM 31: 9-10,14-15a

Be gracious to me, O Lord, for I
am in distress;
my eye is wasted from grief,
my soul and my body also.
For my life is spent with sorrow,
And my years with sighing;
and my strength fails because of my misery,
and my bones waste away . . .

But, I trust in thee, O Lord,
I say, "Thou art my God."
My times are in thy hand;

This passage is particularly helpful during the earlier stages of grief in which the person can identify with feelings and sorrow. There is no need to say more about the depletion that one feels when grief is so intense, or continues at this intensity, over a longer period of time. The corresponding reality and imagery is sufficient. When used in a motivational manner, it is the last part that helps people reorganize and face changes. This kind of scripture relies on trust in God as motivator. From this stance, a person can be encouraged to make changes from a faith standpoint. However, there is still a need to learn and practice new things during reorganization, and in recovery. This learning phase can be called the use of talents that God has provided. These talents may shift according to God's plan or the inspiration and insight that a person receives throughout life.

PSALM 137: 1-2,4 AND PSALM 138: 7a, 8a

By the waters of Babylon,
there we sat down and wept, when we remembered
Zion.
On the willows there we hung up our lyres . . .

How shall we sing the Lord's song in a foreign
land?

Though I walk in the midst of trouble,
Thou dost preserve my life;
Thou dost stretch out thy hand . . .

The Lord will fulfill his purpose for me;
Thy steadfast love, O Lord, endures for ever.

This psalm is motivational because of its ability to relate to the present and bridge the future. It can be helpful for those who have been in the depressive and sorrowing stage and are now, in the latter part of that stage, sorting and sifting through the loss. At this point, they are likely to be beginning to experience a more profound understanding and acceptance that their world has changed. Conversely, the passage is not so helpful during denial and intense anger.

In this passage, God is comforter as well as director of the future that includes the grieving person. In this case, God is not only trustworthy, but compassionate and loving. This is what the grieving person needs. Stability is possible through faith in God, rather than through reliance on other relationships or things that change. Plus, the extra gift of this passage is the fact that people can sing (be purposeful) in the midst of some pretty horrendous stuff. The gentle query of "How will you live your life now that this has happened?" (in this foreign land) is a core question. When asked in a timely manner, in the midst of a caring relationship, the question answers the need that the person has—to know if anyone truly understands his or her predicament and spiritual protest.

ECCLESIASTES 1: 17-18

And I applied my mind to know wisdom
and to know madness and folly.
I perceived that this also is but a striving after wind.

For in much wisdom is much vexation,
and he who increases knowledge increases sorrow.

It is difficult for people who have had significant and multiple losses to understand through the wisdom of their mind, why these things have happened to them. They fear moving on without satisfactory answers because the same thing might happen all over again. They no longer know what they thought they knew. In cases of betrayal and horrendous actions or human evil, they do not really trust their senses, and often they protest about God's reasoning and work. Ecclesiastes rightfully addresses the move from innocence to complexity. In some cases, this move does increase sorrow in the sense that one can never be without the experience, and the knowledge, gained during grief. This passage helps people move on, even when their grief work is not all finished and wrapped up in a package with a bow. After all, this life is our life.

ISAIAH 51: 11

And the ransomed of the Lord shall return,
and come to Zion with singing;
everlasting joy shall be upon their heads:
they shall obtain joy and gladness;
and sorrow and sighing shall flee away.

People need to know that recovery is possible. Life can go on, and even be good, and occasionally better. Thus, Isaiah is a helpful motivator. However, do not use this passage with those who have been through horrendous events, such as the holocaust or for those who have lost children. Instead, go back to psalm 31 or 137-138. But, a very painful loss of a job can result in something better down the road. One can recover from the ending of a marriage. Again, the timing of this passage is important. It is perhaps best used to encourage people who are already in the process of reorganizing and need encouragement to learn new things and make better choices.

Spiritual-Survivor Motivators

This cluster of motivators refers to experiences of self-spirit that are internal and perhaps not connected to transcendent or organized religious/spiritual beliefs. In this area, people are often motivated by self-determination, a desire to succeed, an instinctual survivor spark, or factors that define themselves as people who get through difficult times somehow. Interior spirit motivators are often very idiosyncratic. Thus, it is often hard to define the interior spark that motivates each person to face change.

Individuals whose spirits become motivated during loss are often those who have faced multiple losses, survived, and have faith in themselves. Their stories are often difficult to hear. Their successes at making changes are often difficult to describe or to identify in predictable patterns. One common theme is that at some point there was no other choice but to change. The threat of not changing was that of loss of self. For these people, the choice did not appear as a choice. They do what they have to do.

As one woman shared: "I am in a quiet place because I now realize that I cannot keep living the way I have been living. I have to make changes. This is difficult for me. All these years I have lived the way I have because I have had to live this way. I look back and I realize that some of my choices may have been better than others. But I did the best I could, and like you said, I survived. But now, I need to learn new things and make new choices. I need to do it. I know that. I'm just taking a break for a moment before I start the work ahead."

Another man declares that he has no choice but to go forward. Something in him has changed and he knows that his heart is shriveled and that he has lived too long in sorrow. The other day, when he was looking at the sky, he felt called to make changes. He believes that he could learn to trust in himself and that something in him would help guide him on his new path.

Relational Motivators

The two most common motivators to make major changes are personal and transcendent relationships. The will to reorganize is deeply akin, subconsciously, to the will to live. People who have mental illnesses that tend to thwart the will to live, say time and again that they don't kill themselves because of their children, parents, or grandparents. They are haunted by the effect that suicide would have on these relatives. Note that significant others, partners, spouses, friends are not necessarily included in the list of those who typically keep people from acting on suicidal ideation. The other reason given is that suicide is forbidden by God and the church and might lead to eternal damnation, however that is formulated.

These two relationships, personal and transcendent, also motivate people to recover from significant loss. This is true even in conflicted or ambivalent relationships. In the following poem, written four months after my foster mother's death, my grief is borne because of the memories of the way she changed my life. Although her time was brief, and our time certainly had its ups and downs in the early years, she was truly my mother and my friend.

SHE ASKED FOR ME

She asked for me when I was
little—almost ten and drifting
through the summer grasses
waiting to go home.

Yet, she and all her
vision whisked me away
instead to parts unknown
and took me in.

From the beginning she wanted
to teach and I suppose, now
thinking, I wanted to learn
or so it seems.

About strawberries and
raspberries and Arabs
around and swimming away
in watery pools provided.

She also asked for me when
nightmares came and clouds
of dark overtook both she
and then me.

Those were not the sweetest
sounds and new nightmares
gathered in my closet and
in hers grew too.

She never left her homelessness
or mother dead so early and
on this we separated and I now
turn toward healing.

She did not ask for me, when
last her system did shut down
for she did not accept that
she was going.

It was for her I asked when she
was dying and drifting
through the summer grasses
waiting to go home.

People are motivated by even the most conflicted relationships. In some cases, a deceased parent or partner can provide the motivation to move through grief. It is common for persons to realize or project that the deceased person is looking after them in spirit, or would have wanted them to recover. In many cases, the conclusions of the sorting and sifting time can be used to bring strength to the period of reorganization. In some cases, a relationship may have an oppositional effect. People can be motivated to move on and try new things just to show someone that they can do it. Usually there is nothing wrong with this motivator. In fact, it can be powerful.

Social Motivators

Social and cultural influences can also motivate a person to make changes. Social motivators are not as strong as other motivators, but in cases of severely complicated grief they can be helpful when high value is placed on communal and cultural cohesiveness. Cultural and social influences can complicate normal grieving responses, but they can also contain or hold certain behaviors and encourage appropriate (albeit sometimes stereotypical) changes. Social and cultural motivators are indeed complex and often difficult to determine as to their effect on efforts to move toward reorganization.

Iris was brought up in an upper class protestant family. She attended an exclusive school and had all the benefits that such affluence offered. She had been taught that such blessings brought responsibility. Some of that responsibility involved setting an example for others to follow. Her work was to help others and be good people. There were ways of living that just were not suitable to a person of her class and heritage.

However, when her mother died, Iris fell apart. She could no longer function well in her daily life and certainly could not work. Within three years, Iris had become separated from the rest of her family and was homeless and penniless. Any inheritance that had been set aside was tied up in ways to limit her access to it. The rest had already been spent. Iris lived on the street and in shelters that were available to homeless people. As her situation became less and less tenable, Iris found herself in need of more and more help.

One night, Iris found a bottle of pills at the shelter that she was currently living in and took them all. She was found and rushed to the emergency room of the nearest hospital. From there, she was sent to the psychiatric unit and diagnosed with clinical depression. She was placed on antidepressant medication and received some group and individual therapy. Following her hospitalization, Iris was placed in a group home and received follow-up therapy as an outpatient.

Iris remembers well the day she decided to change her life. She was walking down the hall of the clinic to see her therapist and stopped briefly to go to the bathroom. There in the bathroom, she paused to look at herself in the mirror. At first she was appalled at what she saw. She cried. But she continued to look at herself in the mirror. Then she burst into laughter and declared to herself and the mirror, "By god, you've survived, so you might as well put your life back together." This was the first day of a long and arduous reorganization process. One year later, she was in a small apartment with a job and a modest income. On Mother's Day she called her sister. She was doing fine.

Time and Healing

How do you describe the sorting out on arriving at Auschwitz, the separation of children who see a father or mother going away, never to be seen again? How do you express the dumb grief of a little girl and the endless lines of women, children and rabbis being driven across the Polish or Ukrainian landscapes to their deaths? No, I can't do it. And because I'm a writer and teacher, I don't understand how Europe's most cultured nation could have done that. For these men who killed with sub-machine-guns in the Ukraine were university graduates. After-wards they would go home and read a poem by Heine. So what happened? (Wiesel, 1996, # 64210)

Elie Wiesel, author and survivor of the concentration camps, speaks of being on the edge of life and of the continuing impact of the Holocaust:

There isn't a day, there simply isn't a day without my thinking of death or of looking into death, darkness, or seeing that fire or trying to understand what happened. There isn't a day. I don't write about it. I don't speak about it. I try not to touch the subject at all, but it is present. (Wiesel, 1988, p. 246)

Many people say that time heals all things. Give it time. This too shall pass. The truth of these sentiments actually depends on what we put into time. Grief therapy has brought with it the gift of understanding that when time is filled with specifically selected memories, then it can indeed bring healing. The memories need to be rich, diverse, important, small, ordinary, and even colorful, if they are to be carried through time. Painful memories are important too. Time that is filled with memories has its own energy. This energy is the foundation on which hope and healing thrive. During reorganization, an individual has the benefit of having allotted sufficient time to earlier stages of the grieving process. Giving oneself time to grieve is a powerful motivator to undertake the task of reorganization and recovery.

DECISIONS TO MOVE AHEAD

Some people say that once they experienced a need to move on and leave acute grief behind they knew that they would do so. In some cases, a person has a thought that comes to mind. The thought can be quite simple and is not usually experienced as momentous. Rather, it is ordinary, such as, "I have no more tears. I can't live like this. I need to move on."

Practice Decisions

Other people make many practice decisions before the actual decision to leave sorrow and consider reorganization. The difference between a practice decision and one of conviction is recognizable not so much in the actual words as in the tone of voice, a look, or the lack of large muscle movement in the body, or the presence of a small fidgeting movement. Practice decision words usually include an introduction of qualifiers, the passive structure of sentences, a third-person tense, or false motivator words such as "should." At times, practice decisions are quoted as phrases or clichés that the person has heard and is trying to take in, but is not yet able to do so with inner conviction. For example, Gina's practice decision to reorganize often went like this. "I know I should stop grieving Aaron's death and get on with my life, somehow." This she would say while looking at her lap and moving her hands slowly, one over the other.

The Internal Decision

In some cases, a decision to go on is made because a person thinks he or she has a sense of what's ahead. Thus, the decision is made with one foot in the door of the next stage. However, it is also possible for a person to make an internal decision to move before having a sense of what the movement will look like. In this case, the decision may not have enough force to make it obvious to others. For this reason, it may not be possible to determine whether a firm decision has been made without inquiry into internal processes. This is why it is important to pay attention to behavior, verbalizations, and to encourage nonverbal and creative expressions that may indicate change. In the following poem, intense feelings culminate with the internal decision to "let it be." Thus, a decision to stop and rest from the struggle becomes the making of the larger decision to move on toward reorganization and recovery.

DRY THERE IS

Dry
there is and no more
my soul cannot open
the door
to let the gentle
wind inside.

Mended
now the walls of time
and etched forever
way up high.

Now I reach
to find what's stored
for me
midst ill enlightened
eternity.

Strings
no longer hold
the seam
now bonded
by tape once pressed.

A child
and now a woman grown
barely struggling
to hold
the rest.

Let
it be,
I say
to she.

Occasionally, the decision to reorganize actually formulates itself
after some attempts have been made to adapt and change. When this

happens, these are not practice attempts at decision making, but true authentic attempts that require renewed conviction of purpose. Decisions to move ahead are renewed and adapted during reorganization, just as stages of grief are revisited throughout the grief process. Usually, this revisiting process results in refinement and increased focus. Sometimes, the motivating factor for the decision changes, partially, or entirely, leading to a potentially better outcome.

Externalization of the Decision

At some point, other people see the manifestations of a decision to recover from grief. However, only the grieving individual truly knows that he or she has decided to move forward. Only the individual knows the strength of that conviction and what motivates him or her to do so. But, sooner or later, the decision to reorganize will affect one's symptomatic behavior, relationships, and environment.

Yet, it is helpful for internal decisions to be verbalized, or evident, in ways that others can identify and support. The support and resources that come with change become crucial to successful recovery. Thus, therapeutic and caring professionals do well to explore the nature or essence of any decision to move forward. Exploration of this process will aid in solidifying meaningful decisions and working through tentative ones until they have a corresponding internal connection. In some cases, practicing coming up with reasons to move on and choosing hypothetical motivators is very helpful.

Faith and Determination

Faith is not just a religious term. It refers to spirit in action. Faith, in this sense, is just as active as determination. As verb, faith carries, within the decision, a power to move forward into the future. This is because faith is energy that is born within life and therefore promotes life. Faith brings the decision to reorganize to life.

Faith, in this sense, does not refer to teachings, but to worldviews; the embracing of cosmic mystery, and our ability to act powerfully in it. Faith is the active arm of personal spirit. The added benefit of having faith is that there is a self-rewarding mechanism built into its energy system that reinforces decisions that promote life. Reflection on actions taken through faith energies, is also rewarding. Thus, therapy and spiritual care exercises are doubly helpful in that these processes promote faith/determination and reward actions taken in good faith. In the poem below, the effects of faithful reflection are affirmed many years after a significant and painful loss.

STRONGER

stronger for being alone,
feeling not the touch barely grazing
the cheek, unshed tears of disconnection,
knowing not what is going on, but feeling
so intensely—lost

stronger for thinking within,
wondering with creativeness throughout
the external work of academia,
not just allotted, but declared good, as in
gifts identified—found

stronger for being able to
woman the distance, not knowing
the difference anymore between connection
and disconnection, being and was, not
quite grown—but stronger.

Hope and Future

Hope and future are inextricably intertwined. According to the playwright and politician Vaclav Havel,

> Hope is definitely not the same thing as optimism. It is not the conviction that something will turn out well, but the certainty that something makes sense, regardless of how it turns out. (Havel, 1990, p. 181)

Many people who have been through significant trauma and grief would agree with this definition of hope as not dependent on a conviction that something will turn out well. Some experiences do not have happy endings where everyone feels good. However, it may not be true that hope contains the certainty that something makes sense, or that one can use reason, or sound thinking, to make sense out of events.

Hope is not a convincing thought, or feeling, rather it is the genuine experience of a reality that is—and moves us into the future.

This is the essence of hope in recovery. Some things don't work out well, or at least not to our satisfaction. Some losses don't make sense, yet they are losses from which we must recover, through the process of hoping that the future is coming our way. What may make sense may not be at all related to the loss. For these reasons, one can sometimes displace one's focus on other more important hopes. In many cases, displacement and redirection leads to meaningful paths that might otherwise not have been taken. The following poem speaks of the spirit action of changed direction that is born through the process of hope.

ODE TO DREAMS

Come forth unbidden that you are
'neath the lazy clouds of vision.
Speak to me in other shades
once given over to apple trees
and farming ways.

Lazy days and sweet ambitions,
midst touches strong and tender.
Sometimes darkness, lurking
fears, and memories abounding.

Come forth you. Comfort. Once
unknown now a part of mine
is woven. All that was and might
have been, in truth and fantasy,
my chosen.

Destiny at this late stage,
spoke out and changed direction.
No more paths, of was and whence,
wind round my space now
filled with boundless vision.

CHALLENGES TO REORGANIZATION

Reorganization entails numerous challenges. Some of these challenges are part of the normal grief process and sometimes become complications that lead to dysfunctional responses. Thus, it is important not to assume that because a person is making changes that he or she is out of the proverbial woods. One can be just as vulnerable during reorganization as during previous grief stages.

In fact, a personal and spiritual woundedness can develop during reorganization that is more akin to narcisstic woundedness. Therefore, the anger and intermittent depression that can follow frustrations at this stage can be quite problematic. This is because the self is gaining purposeful momentum. Obstacles during reorganization are perceived as additional losses.

The challenges listed below are often part of the potential factors that place a person at risk for not completing tasks that are essential to reorganization, and having unresolved grief residue that affects recovery and approaches to later losses.

Anniversaries and Reminders

It is common to remember important dates and significant associations throughout one's life. This alone does not make grief complicated or dysfunctional. However, in severely complicated grieving, people frequently find themselves experiencing symptoms and behaviors that continue to arise surrounding these seminal events.

In Amy's case, all would be going well until the anniversary of her mother's death. For one month before this anniversary, she would become pensive, moody, and lethargic. Upon reflection, she would realize that her mother's death anniversary was coming up, but there was nothing she could do. At least six weeks out of the year, she would need to take an antidepressant and live with the fact that she was not functional during this time. Friends said she shouldn't continue to suffer so. After all, it had been almost a dozen years since her mother had passed away. It didn't seem reasonable to them. Her mother had been almost ninety, had had a good life, and died peacefully in her sleep. Still, those six weeks were very problematic for Amy, and for all those who cared about her.

Amy needed therapy. Because she functioned so well during the rest of the year, she might be a candidate for behavioral therapy to help manage these weeks better. She certainly should make some attempt to find out what meaning these six weeks had for her grief process, and perhaps problem solve how her current behaviors fit in with her present life, and what other losses might have piggybacked onto the initial loss of her mother.

High-Risk Thinking

High-risk thinking is any kind of thinking that causes individuals to set up situations that put them at risk. Often, this thinking is disguised as part of an illness, or disorder, or part of a change that is touted as exciting and unrelated to a loss. High-risk thinking requires therapeutic intervention if the behaviors that result are life threatening or escalate over time. Because a person may or may not be aware of thinking patterns, it may be difficult to confront such thinking in a way that will lead to modification and insight. Unlike high-risk thinking, at earlier stages this type of thinking during reorganization is best confronted by going back to the decision-making process that immediately precedes attempts to reorganize. In some instances, one will find that this process was somehow flawed. The reasons for the initial decision to move on may be negative or be motivated by retaliatory gain. External pressures may have coerced the decision. Thus, there is no true energy, hope, or faith action that belongs authentically to the person to drive his or her efforts.

Self-Talk Back Talk

Productive processes engaged during reorganization are usually dependent on positive thinking and feedback that is encouraging, perhaps occasionally ambivalent, but generally supportive. However, during complicated and dysfunctional grief responses, a lingering negative feedback loop may be set in place. This negative loop may seem to be connected to a current moment, but in reality, has become a habitual inner conversation that has the flavor of oppositional thinking, and is under the guise of rational thinking. When this is the case, the person is at odds with self and sabotages his or her efforts to recover.

Because the language of self-talk is so familiar to self, often brief therapeutic interventions are needed that focus on restructuring thinking patterns and inserting more positive thinking processes. Sometimes, all that is needed is to have the person go to a bookstore and find resources in the self-help section. This form of self-help, and self-correction, is only useful for the highly motivated person who is mature enough to observe samples of his or her own thinking patterns and has sufficient desire to make changes.

Sinking Moments

During reorganization, sinking moments are to be expected. However, those who are recovering from complicated and dysfunctional grief responses may fear that sinking moments are signs that they are going back into earlier stages of grief. Thus, the sinking moment may feel like an additional loss and bring about anticipatory grief responses that may be greater than the current small moment would warrant.

In truth, sinking moments, during reorganization, are often mini attempts to sort and sift through the original loss, having gained some distance. Therapeutic interventions may or may not be needed. Recurrent sinking moments that are unmanageable are of course cause for consultation. Otherwise, the best therapeutic intervention is to prepare the person for this process ahead of time and practice problem solving and coping techniques. As indicated in the poem below, it is important not to minimize, or globalize, these sinking moments. Rather, empathize with the person that these moments may be excruciating mini capsules of full-blown grief that is waning.

TATTERED-WHOLENESS

Depths of now
would mean going
below, behind, cold

stuffy nose and
scratchy throat to
find spirit which
is huddled together
at cellular level
to fight invaders.
Tattered-wholeness
like a small dog
nipping at one's ankles.

Unfinished Business

To a certain degree, there is always unfinished business in our lives. However, in complicated and dysfunctional grief responses, the unfinished business is not just a minor challenge. It becomes a major obstacle to recovery. This is so because enough grief has to be re-solved to free a person to reorganize his or her life. Some unfinished business can be resolved though self-reflective processes such as journaling, artistic expressions, and poetry, as seen in the poem below.

MY NAME ISN'T THERE

My name isn't there.
I shouldn't have looked,
nor wondered, nor wished,
for just an ordinary notation
to confirm an importance needed
so intensely as time goes by
and life becomes but simple doings.

No word remains
on tongue nor scrawled across
expanse of white, stiff and fragile,
addressed in person
from our midst, like tall ships
once gone to sea but now returned,
emptied of stores from which to share.

Condemned to fly faceless
through the universe showing up
among the plentitude of summer days,
struggling to remain through depths of cold.
Now caught in winter's attic of the soul
for lack of mirror, of wings, and time,
and wishes bold.

At other times, unfinished business may provide the impetus for professional care and treatment. Reorganization may be the perfect time to undertake insightful therapy because the person is often experiencing an increase in motivation and in energy. Particularly helpful at this time are therapeutic efforts to increase one's capacity to grow and develop personal meaning and connective relationships.

Resistance to Change

One of the changes that tends to be resisted is the integration of undesired thoughts and feelings that have emerged due to the grieving process. Certain thoughts and feelings are resisted even during the reorganization phase, bringing denial temporarily back into the process. Initial denial mechanisms protect an individual from the impact of a loss. During this stage, denial acts as a cushion to contain the effects of that initial experience. Later on, denial has the same kind of effect. It also attempts to slow down changes in self-understanding. Denial is usually a modulating mechanism that often serves a useful purpose in the long run.

To use resistance therapeutically and caringly, it must be understood for its content, timing, and helpfulness to the person. Generally, resistance can be seen as a door that connects people to that which is important to them. For example, a bright, caring, creative woman might want to resist changing her understanding of herself as being a positive individual. She may resist the very idea that she is seething with anger and extremely angry with her spouse, with whom she feels highly competitive and desirous of controlling. To integrate these aspects of herself, she would have to enlarge her self-image to incorporate a new understanding that includes wider aspects of her personality. This she could do, were she to use the grief that has come her way during a painful separation and consequent depression.

Chronic Illness

We have talked about how chronic illness is a complicating factor in the grief process. When chronic illness results in a semipermanent loss of health, reorganization may involve a whole new worldview, and the development of skills that are quite different from those required by less catastrophic losses. To reorganize while in the midst of chronic illness is truly challenging. On these occasions, it is always wise to encourage persons to learn as much as possible about the illness, and to remember that they may not have a choice about their illness, but they are never without choice. It is their responsibility to make the choices they have. This type of supportive confrontation is often possible during the reorganization stage, after a decision to move on has occurred.

Bad Habits

Bad habits, within the framework of loss and recovery, are either responses to loss, or stress responses, or they indicate uncompleted developmental tasks. However, not all bad habits are equal. Thus, it is best not to change some habits until issues that threaten safety and functioning have been addressed. It is helpful to encourage a person to list all the changes that he or she thinks need to be addressed and then problem solve strategies to examine these issues in a somewhat orderly manner over time. Some bad habits, such as smoking and overeating, are best tackled in group therapy and support groups.

Addictions

Addictions are best referred to programs specifically designed for the purposes of recovery from addiction. In some cases, it is appropriate for the person to immerse him or herself in this kind of program prior to other treatment. Sometimes, other therapies may be used to get the person into the contemplation stage of recognizing addiction. By all means never ignore an addiction. At the same time, pay attention to family members and significant others. Although an addiction belongs to a specific person, the addiction has control of the whole relational system. The development of spiritual resources is crucial to recovery from addiction, and may be a component in a recovery program, or an additional adjunct therapy.

Relational Turmoil

To be connected, or not, is really no longer a choice. This is what is recognized during recovery. The interconnectedness of all is essential for healing, wholeness, and recovery. Yet, our natural tendencies are challenged by torn connections, frozen connections, false connections, weak connections, and improper connections. Illness, for example, is a sure indicator of a challenged connection.

Relational turmoil can be considered a normal part of life for some people. While this kind of distorted relationship is something that some people live with, it is not an inevitable part of life, particularly when it exists on a grand scale. The challenge one faces, when assessing relational turmoil, is to identify the intensity and risk of such turmoil to each member of the relationship and to the relational system as a whole.

Relational turmoil is not always bad. Sometimes, relational turmoil is the conduit through which creative change occurs. The greater the change that is required, the greater the potential for turmoil. Thus, turmoil can be normalized as a component of change, and coping methods can be taught to handle the effects of this turmoil. One of the realities of reorganization, after significant loss, is that some additional relationships are lost as a result of the initial loss. Others are transitory. Transitory losses bring their own painful grief process as demonstrated in the following poem.

THE BRIGHT OF DAY

> I can't go there anymore
> for I am scared of what I'll find,
> or not, as it were,
> and in truth it hurts to touch.
> Like grasping tongs of steel,
> once heated by fire now smoldering,
> I jump away in pain.

Yet, I remember deep in my soul,
some need, some desire
that once was kindled,
in a more caring and gentle way.
And I worked on that,
building bridges, where I thought
friendship grew and blossomed.

And now, I wonder. Unhooked
as we are, did we just fill time,
knowing how to be no other.
Did you put up with me
and I, desperate dreamer that I am,
weave with strand and shuttle,
gossamer out of more thin air.

The truth, now whispered in voice
grown dim, I've lost my way.
And there's no one reaching back to me,
no hands where once have been,
no paths to travel, nor uncharted places
calling from within, nor breaks to
shield the bright of day.

Carrying Grief Throughout Life

It is certainly a challenge to grieve and to become a person who needs to hold grief through time. The best way to approach this challenge is to respect a person whose grief response is so profound that it becomes part of the fabric of who he or she is from this time forward. Lasting grief has its own transforming process that brings grace and dignity to the people within which it resides. This kind of grief with its transforming nature can have a positive effect on those whose lives are related to it. When there is not a transforming nature to this kind of grief, then it is rightly termed chronic grief and may be a bereavement disorder or illness in its own right. As illness, it requires sophisticated treatment interventions. As transforming process, it requires creative outlet.

DEVELOPING A LIFELONG HABIT OF LEARNING

Life has its own way of encouraging us to learn and grow. Sometimes we find the learning process engaging, pleasant, and creative. At other times we learn the hard way. I grew up in a family of educators, so learning was often more important than anything else. For our family, academic education was a god to which we never paid enough homage. We were not encouraged to learn as much about psychological and spiritual challenges as we were about getting degrees and amounting to something in the vocational market. It was not until I neared the completion of a doctoral program, in which I specialized in treatment for trauma and grief, did I really come to know a corresponding love of learning. Therefore, I pass along my most significant piece of learning to you: Take time to love life and to love learning about all of life. Then, take time to understand loss and to treasure relationships.

One year before my first book on grief education was published, I realized that I had not done what I intended to do in terms of recording, through poetry, the lives of some 100-plus elders in a nursing home. When I realized this, they were discharged to other places or had long since received a celestial discharge to heaven. I had to adapt my plans and devise a way to place closure on those relationships. The following poem is about what I learned, in a painful and humbling way.

I THOUGHT THERE WOULD BE TIME

Looking over my notes
from years ago
I find names and notations
of 107 elderly residents who were,
in my mind,
going to be the 100 eyes
in poetic renderings.

Most are gone now
maybe forty remain
a few are still to be mentioned.

There were comments.
"I want to die."
"I thought you'd like to know."
"Not bad for 94."

And there were
the deaf
the blessed with sight
the blind
those with arthritis
those with cancer
and broken hips

And questions!
"Where's the church?"
"Where have you been?"
"Lunch, Dear?"

There were relatives . . .
husbands
sisters
mothers
sons
and
daughters

Believers and unbelievers . . .
Baptists
Catholics
those with no stock in religion
TV preacher watchers
doxology singers
candle lighters
memories of church and mother
memorized prayer and high-pitched verses

And those on the move . . .
with working hands
driving Caddies
walking and smoking

and wandering
doing needlework
flinging arms and feet
and pulling stitches

And those restrained . . .
in beds
in chairs
lying down
alone
and lost
young and stranded

And there were the colorful . . .
all in red
pink and lovely
staring in mirrors
wearing Sunday hats
all dressed up and where to go?

And many relational . . .
giving hugs
singing tunes
acting coy
bringing kisses
holding fuzzies
mimicking words
and sharing "hi"s

Feeling pains . . .
moans and groans
quiet fears and little comforts
gruff and gruffer
hating holidays
weathering the bad days

Getting help . . .
smiles and hair strokes
candy and visits

holding on
reading *Playboy* and getting religion
welcoming sleep
and giving it a try
watching sports
reading poetry
playing the harmonica and violin
and remembering the farm

Looking over my notes
from years ago
I find names and notations
on 107 elderly residents who were,
in my mind,
going to be the 100 eyes
in poetic renderings
so I would always remember.

I thought there would be time.

Do not be afraid to present what you have learned from your own experience and the experience of working with others. Letting a person know that you have heard similar responses can sometimes be reassuring. A woman who had multiple tragic events in her life including divorce and lost custody of her teenager, had this to say: "I thought I was the only one who felt this way. I thought my problems happened because I was weak. I thought that post-traumatic stress disorder was just for those who have been in combat. I guess not. I guess it happens to many people. It helps me to know that and to hear that there is effective treatment." While not disclosing any specifics about others, it is quite possible to affirm common responses and issues.

Do not be afraid to talk about life with colleagues, and to share from your experience, and the experience of working with others. Do not be afraid to frame things humanely, ethically, and with spirit. This is how you develop your personal style and the uniqueness of your work. This is how you can engage in planning for positive outcomes and learn new techniques and strategies to serve people. There is always time to consult and to grow as a professional.

Capacity, Resiliency, and Change

Through a commitment to lifelong learning, and love and respect of all of life, we enlarge our capacity to function well, our resiliency in meeting our own needs and the needs of others, and our capacity to change and become change agents in a world that thrives on flux. Some people call the context of our relational life the web of life. It is an apt image. Nowhere is it more imperative to find our way through this marvelous, tenuous, and vulnerable web, than it is during a period of loss and grief. We coach, teach, and become bearers of the meaning of life only as we are able to network with those we work with, live with, and professionally help. As indicated in the following poem, nothing is too ordinary to be noticed. No one is too ordinary to be a resource for our own growth and development in the very ordinary and complex world of working with those in the midst of grief.

NETWORKING

Moving softly this morning
midst thoughts of change
watching sky blue wires
laid outside my door to catch
the words the women type
and send them across the
byways of sound. Energy
in and energy out, and
so it goes, goes, goes.

In this round storage
system I call my mind
the wires are so intertwined
I wonder with early risings
where to send what, to whom
and how to command one
thought in the midst of many
or check random feelings
and long-ago messages

that have no time. And
so it goes, goes, goes.

RECLAIMING LIFE

Reclaiming one's life after a loss is a heroic affair. There is nothing grandiose about this claim. Rather the magnitude of what people face in life is often beyond what anyone ever imagines. Each person's story is filled with a pathos that would often defy the originators of classical Greek tragedy. However, professionals and other helpers who provide care in such circumstances have proverbial feet of clay and are often armed solely by their compassion and their desire to promote healing. The companionship of such a pair, the wounded hero and the compassionate but ordinary professional caregiver, are essential to reclaiming a life that may be losing its way. The task on the wounded hero's part is nothing but essential. The task on the caregiver's part is surely folly. Yet together, healing happens.

In Lieu of a Magic Wand

Michael came to the loss and recovery group and sat with his arms crossed over his chest. He was a short, middle-aged man of slight build who wore a baseball cap pulled tightly over his head and skin-tight jeans. When it was his turn to speak, he stated that he had been in the hospital for two weeks. He was being discharged and it was incredible, for the hospital had done nothing for him.

He was losing weight. He stood and raised his shirt up to his armpits showing off an emaciated rib cage. He stated, "Does this look normal to you?" Following that, he sat down and continued, with his frustration now directed at this "class," saying that this was his second time and the class was doing nothing for him. When asked what problems he had that he felt weren't being addressed, he listed multiple problems. He said the doctor had told his mother that she needed to cut the apron strings. He thought his mother was doing what a mother should do. He said he had a mood disorder, PTSD, was an alcoholic with liver damage, had an eating disorder, and had been sexually molested as a child.

Sometimes, the only answer is that loss and grief never seem to end. Michael felt that he never gets a chance to get out of shock, denial, and anger. Care, kindness, and empathy were all I had to offer, along with a psychoeducational approach to helping him develop some understanding of what he was going through, and of the concerted long-term efforts that he had to make for things to improve. This effort was something that was his to do, or not do, whether as outpatient or inpatient.

Michael listened closely to others who were angry about being hospitalized. About twenty minutes later, he quietly said, "I don't think I'm so much angry as I am disappointed." This was the moment Michael decided to work. He could do this because the therapist had affirmed his situation, his grief story, his feelings, and indicated that she knew something about the grief process that he was going through. The therapist responded with, "It makes sense that you feel disappointed. Under that feeling you are probably a little afraid." To this he nodded his head in the affirmative.

On my way back to the office, I felt some of Michael's grief burden. While grabbing a bowl of soup, I found myself thinking, "Gee whiz, June, this was session number two, and you haven't fixed the problem yet! Where is your magic wand?" Then I realized that this remains the real spiritual dilemma in severely complicated grief. If Jesus could heal all people, why was he so stingy about it? Of course, I told myself that if I had the power, I would be more than happy to heal everyone. This is when I realized that, in lieu of a magic wand, the power I had was caring, kindness, and empathy along with an ability to approach the situation with some knowledge and growing skill. In a way, all this was magical and miraculous for Michael who for once felt heard, and stepped that day into a new relationship.

May you bless others with caring companionship on their grief journeys!

Appendix A

Universal Grief Response

Attachment—Close connectedness to people who are important in one's life

Shock—Physiological response (eyes open wider, jaw drops slightly)

Denial—Protective response that modulates feelings/thoughts that come later

Feelings—Sadness, fear, anger, regret, and many more

Depression—A comprehensive sorting process that normally culminates with a sense of a need to "go on"

Reorganization—The learning or skill phase of recovery that focuses on changes in one's life as a result of the loss

Recovery—Making new attachments and investing more energy in ongoing relationships

Note: See also McCall (1999) 41-62.

Appendix B

Possible Complications
Surrounding Significant Loss

GRIEF STAGES

Shock/Denial

- Actual difficulty processing that a death or major loss has occurred
- Initial denial of magnitude of the loss
- Inability to observe societal rituals surrounding death or significant loss

Feelings

- Managing forbidden grief
- Ambivalent, violent, overpowering, unsanctioned attachments
- Large degree of anger, guilt, and feelings caused by emotional secrets
- Lack in capacity to access, identify, or express feelings

Depression

- Sadness or sorrow that becomes pervasive and remains intense over an extended time
- Lack of ability/success in sorting through/reviewing a relationship
- Problems deciding to move on

Reorganization

- Difficulty learning new skills
- Unwillingness to make necessary changes

Recovery

- Struggles with ongoing relationships
- Diminished/impaired capacity to love again
- Diminished faith/trust in the benevolence of the world/people

Note: See also McCall (1999) 60-61; Rando (1993) 185-240; Sanders (1989) 111-126; Worden (1982) 53-63.

Appendix C

Identification of Risk Factors That May Lead to Complicated and Dysfunctional Grieving

General Factors

- Nature of the relationship
- Nature of the loss
- Physical, psychological, sociological, and spiritual condition of the survivor
- Resources available to the bereaved (McCall, 1999, 49-53)

Particularly at Risk

- Persons with multiple losses
- Persons with extensive loss history—particularly at vulnerable periods
- Persons who have experienced severe trauma
- Persons whose loved one died violent, horrendous, or unfathomable deaths
- Persons with concurrent mental illness—particularly depression and anxiety
- Persons with Axis 2 traits—dependency, borderline, etc.
- Persons who tend to extremes—minimization/maximization
- Persons who are isolated
- Persons contending with "real" guilt
- Persons with major life-skill deficits
- Persons who lose children

Note: See also Rando (1993) 30-33, 453-463, 511-517, 569-571.

Appendix D

Grief Trajectory Worksheet:
Complicated/Dysfunctional Grief

Date_____

Name_____

Loss_____

_____

Brief Loss History_____

_____

_____

_____

Obstacle (problem or impairment)	Locus	Grief Stage	Duration	Severity
1.	Physical Psychological Social Spiritual	Shock Denial Feelings Depression Reorganization Recovery	Temporary Short Term Long Term	Mild Moderate Severe 1 2 3 4 5
2.	Physical Psychological Social Spiritual	Shock Denial Feelings Depression Reorganization Recovery	Temporary Short Term Long Term	Mild Moderate Severe 1 2 3 4 5

3.	Physical Psychological Social Spiritual	Shock Denial Feelings Depression Reorganization Recovery	Temporary Short Term Long Term	Mild Moderate Severe 1 2 3 4 5

Grief Trajectory Template (circle completed stages):

Shock   Recovery

        Denial   Reorganization

                Feelings   Depression

Appendix E

Grief Response Service Wheel

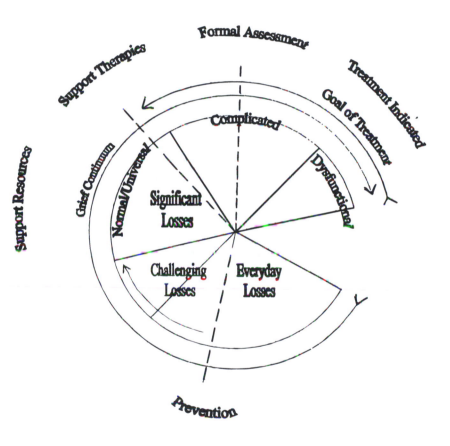

Appendix F

Severity of Grief Response: Impairment Flow Sheet Template

Normal	Mild Complication	Moderate Complication	Severe/ Dysfunctional Responses
Problem			
Problem			
Problem			
Problem			
Stress	More Stress	Distress	Dysfunction/Impairment

Appendix G

Dysfunctional Grieving Criteria: Symptoms and Behavior That Can Indicate Dysfunctional Grieving

1. **Denial of death/loss**
   - After reasonable time
   - When confronted with facts of death
2. **Aggressive, violent, and impulsive behaviors**
   - Perhaps suicidal
   - Not present prior to loss
   - Cannot be attributed to later events
3. **Depression and increasing anxiety**
   - That interferes with normal, essential, daily activities
   - May include apathy or lack of interest and pleasure
4. **Extended assignment of a significant loss as cause for current difficulties**
   - When exploration of that loss does not yield reasonably understandable connections
5. **Lingering spiritual distress or despair**
   - Including existential bitterness
   - Loss of trust, faith, or hope
   - Not present prior to loss
   - Cannot be attributed to later events
6. **Extended withdrawal from relationships that were formerly comforting**
7. **Harmful practices**
   - Use and/or abuse of drugs, alcohol
   - Health threatening overeating/undereating
   - Noncompliance with medications not otherwise attributable to mental illness or prior difficulties
8. **Dependency**
   - Insatiable neediness
   - Diminished initiative and accountability
   - Not attributable to prior difficulties or new health issues

9. **Risk taking**
   - Lack of attention to personal safety
   - Lack of limit setting
   - Challenging of rules and customs
   - Not part of former personality profile
10. **Lingering sense of general foreboding**
    - Regarding future losses that appear to have no rational basis
    - Something clouding the future

Bibliography

Anandarajah, Gowri and Ellen Hight (2001)."Spirituality and Medical Practice: Using the HOPE Questions as a Practical Tool for Spiritual Assessment." *American Family Physician,* 63(1): 81-88.

Antczak, Marianne (1999). "Attending to the Grief Associated with Involuntary Job Loss." *The Journal of Pastoral Care,* 53(4): 447-460.

Barboncito, Navajo Chief at the Signing of The Navajo Treaty —1868 (1968). Las Vegas, NV: K.C. Publications, p. 5.

Barrett, Deborah (1999)."Suffering and the Process of Transformation." *The Journal of Pastoral Care,* 53(4): 461-473.

Bateman, Anne, Dena Broderick, Louise Gleason, Reb Kardon, Cynthia Flaherty, and Susan Anderson (1992). "Dysfunctional Grieving." *The Journal of Psychosocial Nursing,* 30(12): 5-9.

Benson, Herbert (1996). *Timeless Healing: The Power and Biology of Belief.* New York: Scribner.

Benzein, Eva, Astrid Norberg, and Britt-Inger Saveman (1998)."Hope: Future Imagined Reality. The Meaning of Hope As Described by a Group of Healthy Pentecostalists." *The Journal of Advanced Nursing,* 28(5): 1063-1070.

Bonanno, George and Stacey Kaltman (2001)."The Varieties of Grief Experience." *Clinical Psychology Review,* 21(5): 705-734.

Bonhoeffer, Deitrich (1954). *Life Together.* San Francisco: Harper and Row.

Boutell, Karen and Frederick Bozett (1990)."Nurses' Assessment of Patients' Spirituality: Continuing Education Implications." *The Journal of Continuing Education in Nursing,* 21(4): 172-176.

Brabant, Sarah and Mary Martof (1993). "Childhood Experiences and Complicated Grief: A Study of Adult Children of Alcoholics." *The International Journal of the Addictions,* 28(11): 1111-1125.

Brintzen-hofeSzoc, Elizabeth Smith, and James Zabora (1999). "Screening to Predict Complicated Grief in Spouses of Cancer Patients." *Cancer Practice,* 7(5): 233-239.

Brown Taylor, Barbara (1998). *When God Is Silent: The 1997 Lyman Beecher Lectures on Preaching.* Boston: Cowley Publications.

Clinebell, Howard (1992). *Well-Being: A Personal Plan for Exploring and Enriching the Seven Dimensions of Life.* San Francisco: HarperCollins.

Crenshaw, David A. (1990). *Bereavement: Counseling the Grieving Throughout the Life Cycle.* New York: Continuum.

Cressey, R.W. and M. Winbolt-Lewis (2000). "The Forgotten Heart of Care: A Model of Spiritual Care in the National Health Service." *Accident and Emergency Nursing,* 8(3): 170-177.

Cutcliffe, John (1998). "Hope, Counseling and Complicated Bereavement Reactions." *Journal of Advanced Nursing,* 28 (4): 754-761.

Dossey, Larry (1993). *Healing Words: The Power of Prayer and the Practice of Medicine.* New York: HarperCollins.

Easterling, Larry, Louis Gamino, Kenneth Sewell, and Linda Stirman (2000). "Spiritual Experience, Church Attendance, and Bereavement." *Journal of Pastoral Care,* 54(3): 263-276.

Ezzy, Douglas (2000). "Illness Narratives: Time, Hope and HIV." *Social Science & Medicine,* 50(5): 605-617.

Fetzer Institute, National Institute on Aging Working Group (1999). *Multidimensional Measurement of Religiousness/Spirituality for Use in Health Research: A Report of the Fetzer Institute/National Institute on Aging Working Group.* Kalamazoo, MI: John E. Fetzer Institute.

Frank, Arthur (1995). *The Wounded Storyteller: Body, Illness, and Ethics.* Chicago: The University of Chicago Press.

Fry, Virginia (1995). *Part of Me Died, Too: Stories of Creative Survival Among Bereaved Children and Teenagers.* New York: Dutton/Penguin.

Glassman, Bernard and Rick Fields (1996). *Instructions to the Cook: A Zen Master's Lessons in Living a Life That Matters.* New York: Bell Tower.

Harris, Chandice (1984). "Dysfunctional Grieving Related to Childbearing Loss: A Descriptive Study." *Health Care for Women International,* 5: 401-425.

Havel, Vaclav (1990). *Disturbing the Peace.* New York: Alfred A. Knopf.

Hershey, Terry (2000). *Soul Gardening: Cultivating the Good Life.* Minneapolis: Augsburg.

Holy Bible (1972). Revised Standard Version. Nashville: Thomas Nelson Inc.

Horowitz, Mardi, Bryna Siegel, Are Holen, George Bonanno, Constance Milbrath, and Charles Stinson (1997). "Diagnostic Criteria for Complicated Grief Disorder." *American Journal of Psychiatry,* 154(7): 904-910.

Kirkpatrick, Helen, Janet Landeen, Harriet Woodside, and Carolyn Byrne (2001). "How People with Schizophrenia Build Their Hope." *Journal of Psychosocial Nursing and Mental Health Services,* 39(1): 46-53.

Kissane, David, Sidney Bloch, Partick Onghena, Dean McKenzie, Ray Snyder, and David Dowe (1996). "The Melbourne Family Grief Study, II: Psychosocial Morbidity and Grief in Bereaved Families." *American Journal of Psychiatry,* 153(5): 659-666.

Kleindienst, Martha (1998). "Spirituality—Where There Is Hope, There Is Life." *ANNA Journal,* 25(4): 442.

Koenig, Harold (1997). *Is Religion Good for Your Health?* Binghamton, NY: The Haworth Press, Inc.

Kornfeld, Margaret (2000). *Cultivating Wholeness.* New York: Continuum.

Lester, Andrew (1995). *Hope in Pastoral Care and Counseling.* Louisville, KY: Westminster John Knox Press.

Maercker, Andreas, George Bonanno, Hansjoerg Znoj, and Mardi Horowitz (1998). "Prediction of Complicated Grief by Positive and Negative Themes in Narratives." *Journal of Clinical Psychology,* 54(8): 1117-1136.

Marwit, Samuel (1996). "Reliability of Diagnosing Complicated Grief: A Preliminary Investigation," *Journal of Consulting and Clinical Psychology,* 64(3): 563-568.

Mayo, Peg Elliott (2001). *The Healing Sorrow Workbook: Rituals for Transforming Grief and Loss.* Oakland, CA: New Harbinger Publications, Inc.

McBride, J. LeBron (1998). *Spiritual Crisis: Surviving Trauma to the Soul.* Binghamton, NY: The Haworth Press, Inc.

McCall, Junietta (1999). *Grief Education for Caregivers of the Elderly.* Binghamton, NY: The Haworth Press, Inc.

McDermott, Holly Prigerson, Charles Reynolds, Patricia Houck, Mary Drew, Martica Hall, Sati Mazumdar, Daniel Buysse, Carolyn Hoch, and David Kupher (1997). "Sleep in the Wake of Complicated Grief Symptoms: An Exploratory Study." *Biological Psychiatry,* 41: 710-716.

Melhem, Nadine, Carlos Rosales, Jason Karageorge, Charles Reynolds, Ellen Frank, and M. Katherine Shear (2001). "Comorbidity of Axis I Disorders in Patients with Traumatic Grief." *The Journal of Clinical Psychiatry,* 62(11): 884-886.

Merton, Thomas (1990). *Thoughts in Solitude.* (Eighteenth Printing) New York: The Noonday Press, Farrar, Straus and Giroux.

Middleton, Warwick, Paul Burnett, Beverly Raphael and Nada Martinek, (1996). "The Bereavement Response: A Cluster Analysis." *British Journal of Psychiatry* 169: 167-171.

Muller, Wayne (1993). *Legacy of the Heart: The Spiritual Advantages of a Painful Childhood.* New York: Simon and Schuster.

O'Connor, Rory and Noel Sheehy (2001). "Suicidal Behavior." *The Psychologist,* 14(1): 20-24.

O'Connor, Thomas and Elizabeth Meakes (1998). "Hope in the Midst of Challenge: Evidence-Based Pastoral Care." *The Journal of Pastoral Care,* 52(4): 389-396.

Oxford Annotated Bible, Revised Standard Version (1962). New York: Oxford University Press.

Pfeiffer, Joseph and J. Kent Usry (2000). *Bereavement Handouts: Reproducible Educational Handouts for Clients.* Memphis, TN: Landscapes Publishing.

Phillips, Michael, Nicholas Ward, and Richard Ries (1983). "Fictitious Mourning: Painless Patienthood." *American Journal of Psychiatry,* 140(4): 420-425.

Piper, William, Mary McCallum, Anthony Joyce, John Rosie, and John Ogrodniczuk (2001). "Patient Personality and Time-Limited Group Psychotherapy for Complicated Grief." *International Journal of Group Psychotherapy,* 51(4): 525-552.

Piper, William, John Ogrodniczuk, Hassan Azim, and Rene Wiedeman (2001). "Prevalence of Loss and Complicated Grief Among Psychiatric Outpatients," *Psychiatric Services,* 52(8): 1069-1074.

Piper, William, John Ogrodniczuk, Anthony Joyce, Mary MacCullum, Rene Wiedeman, and Hassan Azim (2001). "Ambivalence and Other Relationship Predictors of Grief in Psychiatric Outpatients." *The Journal of Nervous and Mental Disease,* 189(11): 781-787.

Prigerson, Holly, Andrew Bierhals, Stanislav Kasl, Charles Reynolds, M. Katherine Shear, Jason Newsom, and Selby Jacobs (1996). "Complicated Grief as a Disorder Distinct from Bereavement-Related Depression and Anxiety: A Replication Study." *American Journal of Psychiatry,* 153(1): 1484-1486.

Prigerson, Holly, Ellen Frank, Stanislav Kasl, Charles Reynolds, Barbara Anderson, George Zubenko, Patricia Houck, Charles George, and David Kupfer (1995). "Complicated Grief and Bereavement-Related Depression as Distinct Disorders: Preliminary Empirical Validation in Elderly Bereaved Spouses." *American Journal of Psychiatry,* 152(1): 22-30.

Prochaska, James, John Norcorss, and Carlo Diclemente (1994). *Changing for Good: The Revolutionary Program That Explains the Six Stages of Change and Teaches You How to Free Yourself from Bad Habits.* New York: William Morrow and Company, Inc.

Raleigh, Edith and Susan Boehm (1994). "Development of the Multidimensional Hope Scale." *Journal of Nursing Measurement,* 2(2): 155-167.

Rancour, Patrice (1998). "Recognizing and Treating Dysfunctional Grief," *ONF,* 25(8): 1310-1311.

Rando, Therese (1993). *Treatment of Complicated Mourning.* Champaign, IL: Research Press.

Raphael, Beverly (1983). *The Anatomy of Bereavement.* New York: Basic Books Inc.

Rawlins, Ruth Parmelee, Cornelia Beck, and Sophronia Williams (1988). *Mental Health-Psychiatric Nursing: A Holistic Life-Cycle Approach.* St. Louis: Mosby.

Richardson, Robert (2000). "Where There Is Hope, There Is Life: Toward a Biology of Hope." *The Journal of Pastoral Care,* 54(1): 75-84.

Rosenzweig, Andrew, Holly Prigerson, Mark Miller, and Charles Reynolds (1997). "Bereavement and Late-Life Depression: Grief and Its Complications in the Elderly." *Annual Review of Medicine,* 48: 421-428.

Rozario, Loretta (1997). "Spirituality in the Lives of People with Disability and Chronic Illness: A Creative Paradigm of Wholeness and Reconstitution." *Disability and Rehabilitation,* 19(10): 427-434.

Sanders, Catherine (1989). *Grief: The Mourning After: Dealing with Adult Bereavement.* New York: John Wiley & Sons.

Sarah Plain and Tall: Winter's End (1999). Videocassette, DVD, 99 min. Hallmark Home Entertainment.

Sellers, Sandra and Barbara Haag (1998). "Spiritual Nursing Interventions." *Journal of Holistic Nursing,* 16(3): 338-354.

Stone, Howard (1998). "Depression and Spiritual Desolation." *The Journal of Pastoral Care,* 52(4): 359-368.

Szanto, Katalin, Holly Prigerson, Patricia Houck, Lin Ehrenpreis, and Charles Reynolds (1997). "Suicidal Ideation in Elderly Bereaved: The Role of Complicated Grief." *Suicide and Life-Threatening Behavior,* 27(2): 194-207.

Thurman, Howard (1976). *Meditations of the Heart.* Harper & Row (1953): Reprint, Friends United Press: Richmond.

Walker, Alice (1982). *The Color Purple.* Harcourt Brace: New York.

White, Bowen and John MacDougall (2001). *Clinician's Guide to Spirituality,* New York: McGraw-Hill Medical Publishing Division.

Wiesel, Elie (1988). *Writers at Work: The Paris Review Interviews,* Eight Series, George Plimpton (Ed.). New York: Viking.

Wiesel, Elie (1996). *The Columbia World of Quotations,* Quotation number 64210. (Quoted in *Le Monde,* Paris, June 4, 1987).

Wolfelt, Alan (1991). "Toward an Understanding of Complicated Grief: A Comprehensive Overview." *The American Journal of Hospice & Palliative Care,* March/April: 28-30.

Worden, J. William (1982). *Grief Counseling and Grief Therapy:* New York: Springer Publishing Company.

Yahne, Caroline and William R. Miller (2000). "Evoking Hope." In William R. Miller (Ed.), *Integrating Spirituality into Treatment: Resources for Practitioners* (pp. 217-233). Washington, DC: American Psychological Association.

Zeitlin, Susan (2001). "Grief and Bereavement," *Palliative Care,* 28(2): 415-425.

Index